Morton He

Emotiona.

Hi — HAPPY PRE-
BIRTHDAY. TALKED TO
NANCY DENNIS & BELIEVE

THIS WAY OF APPROACH
RELATES TO
JO SHIN DO
THE BEST, nancy

Morton Herskowitz D. O.

Emotional Armoring

An Introduction to
Psychiatric Orgone Therapy

LIT

Bibliographic information published by the Deutsche Nationalbibliothek
The Deutsche Nationalbibliothek lists this publication in the Deutsche
Nationalbibliografie; detailed bibliographic data are available in the Internet at
http://dnb.d-nb.de.

2. Auflage 2008

ISBN 978-3-8258-3555-2

A catalogue record for this book is available from the British Library

© LIT VERLAG Dr. W. Hopf Berlin 2008
Verlagskontakt:
Fresnostr. 2 D-48159 Münster
Tel. +49 (0) 2 51/620 32 - 22   Fax +49 (0) 2 51/922 60 99
e-Mail: lit@lit-verlag.de   http://www.lit-verlag.de

Auslieferung:
Deutschland/Schweiz: LIT Verlag Fresnostr. 2, D-48159 Münster
Tel. +49 (0) 2 51/620 32 - 22, Fax +49 (0) 2 51/922 60 99, e-Mail: vertrieb@lit-verlag.de
Österreich: Medienlogistik Pichler-ÖBZ GmbH & Co KG
IZ-NÖ, Süd, Straße 1, Objekt 34, A-2355 Wiener Neudorf
Tel. +43 (0) 2236/63 535-290, +43 (0) 2236/63 535 - 243, mlo@medien-logistik.at

Distributed in the UK by: Global Book Marketing, 99B Wallis Rd, London, E9 5LN
Phone: +44 (0) 20 8533 5800 – Fax: +44 (0) 1600 775 663
http://www.centralbooks.co.uk/html

Distributed in North America by:

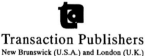

Transaction Publishers
New Brunswick (U.S.A.) and London (U.K.)

Transaction Publishers
Rutgers University
35 Berrue Circle
Piscataway, NJ 08854

Phone: +1 (732) 445 - 2280
Fax: + 1 (732) 445 - 3138
for orders (U. S. only):
toll free (888) 999 - 6778
e-mail:
orders@transactionspub.com

To Karen and Robin

Acknowledgements

Many thanks to Gail Michelle Kemmerer, Ph.D. and to Charlotte Rudnick, Ed.D. for their unstinting efforts in typing the original manuscript, Marcia Sartwell contributed her wise and informed editorial redommendations. To Lillian Somner, D.O. I owe gratitude and admiration for the large amount of work performed in a seemingly effortless manner in preparing the final manuscript and tape. Drs. Dorothea and Manfred Fuckert provided an abundance of energy and time in their effort to achieve publication, a tribute of their friendship. Finally I thank my lucky stars for having brought me into contact with Wilhelm Reich and his work.

Contents

All Bibles or sacred codes have been the cause of the following Errors:

1. *That Man has two real existing principles:*
   Viz: a Body and a Soul.
2. *That Energy, call'd Evil, is alone from the Body;*
   and that Reason, call'd Good, is alone from the Soul.
3. *That God will torment Man in Eternity for following his*
   energies.

But the following Contraries to these are True:

1. *Man has no Body distinct from his Soul; for that call'd Body is a*
   portion of Soul discern'd by the five Senses, the chief inlets of Soul
   in this age.
2. *Energy is the only life, and is from the Body; and Reason is the*
   bound or outward circumference of Energy.
3. *Energy is Eternal Delight.*

William Blake, *The Marriage of Heaven and Hell*

Introduction

A reasonable comprehension of emotional and mental disorder is a relatively recent phenomenon in human history. We have moved through ages where the emotionally afflicted were regarded as devil possessed, victims of curses, paying for sins of past lives and subjects of God's wrath. Consequently, with few exceptions such as the hydrotherapy and music therapy provided by the early Greeks, the treatment of the mentally disabled has been essentially inhumane and isolating. With the ascendance of scientific thought and the diminution of societal superstition there were attempts in the nineteenth century to ameliorate the plight of mental patients. Mesmer introduced the use of hypnosis as a treatment regimen. Rest cures in appealing settings were advocated for those who could afford them. Mental disorder was beginning to be regarded as a province of medicine, a malady to be treated rather than exorcised. Physicians described talking cures as they began to listen to their patients.

Freud's discovery of the unconscious by the process of psychoanalysis marked a phenomenal advance in our awareness of our emotional and mental substance. We learned of motivations formerly unknown for our aberrant behaviors and symptoms. We frequently uncovered sources in traumatic events of early childhood, harvested from previously forgotten memories. Our bizarre behaviors and troubling symptoms were becoming less mysterious.

Unfortunately, though the techniques of psychoanalysis -- free association, dream analysis, slips of the tongue and analysis of resistances -- provided the high road to the discovery of unconscious material, they were far less successful in affording symptomatic relief and significant changes in behavior.

It was not until Wilhem Reich introduced the concept of character analysis into psychoanalysis that more significant therapeutic gains were achieved. Character analysis marked the apogee of Reich's acclaim in the general psychiatric community. From this point on, his creativity soared, his insights were more radical (in the sense of deeply rooted), his mind took more imaginative leaps -- and his reputation within the psychiatric community plummeted. Henceforth, from time to time and from place to place there would be reports of his insanity.

When I was in therapy with Dr. Reich, a friend of mine with distinguished credentials in his medical discipline asked, "What do

7

other psychiatrists think of Reich?" "They all think he's crazy," I answered. When he expressed doubts that level-headed, "top-drawer" professionals shared that view, I challenged him to canvas the members of his school's prestigious psychiatric faculty. He later reported, "Every one of them said that Reich was in an insane asylum and were amazed that I knew someone who was in treatment with him in Forest Hills, New York."

Reich had been one of Freud's inner circle. In time, though, he abandoned psychoanalysis and gradually developed the therapy that is the subject of this book. The beginning point was the recognition that character is rooted in the body as well as the mind. Stubbornness is a stiffness of the back of the neck. Fear is a tightness in the belly. Anger is, in part, a clenching of the jaw. By working to relieve the tension in these armored segments, one is able to reach emotional depths unavailable by talk alone. The relief afforded to patients and the satisfaction to therapists was now significantly enhanced.

With increased experience he developed a stronger theoretical framework for the therapy. He saw that the body's armoring functioned to bind energy; he saw also that the release of the bound energy, especially in large bursts, gave immediate relief but later unease to the individual. He demonstrated that each person's character structure had been shaped so that he could maintain a level of emotional repression that was comfortable for him, even though the repression also reduced his level of energy. Freeing of character structure involved a gradual process of learning to tolerate a higher energy level. And finally Reich became aware that the constrained energy always, in some way, interfered with full orgastic discharge. Our vital energy is our sexual energy. Every living organism is a pulsatile energy system that charges and discharges. The wider the energetic pulsation the more fully that life is lived. Reich's therapeutic prospectus now included, but went beyond psychology into biology and concepts of energy flow.

From here Reich sought to gain elemental energetic insights into basic biological functions, then to discover the physical properties of the energy that infuses us as it exists in the atmosphere at large -- and on and on.

At each new departure those of us who followed Reich would shrink with anxiety. At one such juncture, when I voiced my apprehension in stronger language than necessary, Reich asked, "Haven't I gained any credit with you?"

Reich's ventures into biology, natural science and physics will ultimately (in our lifetime or beyond) be regarded as quantum leaps in scientific thought, or they will be invalidated. What has been true to this point is that those who have worked most seriously to repeat Reich's experimental scientific work are those with whom he has gained the most credit.

He was aware of his effect on less adventurous souls and referred to it as his "too muchness." There is a hope that what is "too much" for us may be right for future generations.

From the perspective of psychiatric orgone therapy (orgone is the name that Reich gave to the energy which moves us), we are descending into a Dark Age in the practice of psychiatry. This, despite the fact that we can relieve 70 percent of depressions with antidepressant drugs, that neuroleptics can ameliorate the hallucinations and delusions of psychotic patients, at least temporarily, that we have solid evidence of the role of genes in some disorders, and that we can pinpoint the metabolic deficit in a specific area of the brain to mark the locus of a particular psychiatric syndrome. The new comprehension of brain chemistry is a remarkable achievement. But rather than becoming an adjunct in treating mental illness, the use of drugs has become an exclusive focus, in psychiatry. The patient is currently looked at as the bearer of symptoms rather than a dynamic, pulsating human being.

But psychiatry started out exploring the immense and fascinating complexity of how we function -- a journey we need to continue. Psychiatry must reach beyond the treatment of isolated symptoms and begin to reveal -- to borrow from literary references -- why we are a "madding crowd" and too often live "lives of quiet desperation." Psychiatric orgone therapy, though it is not a cure-all and though it is not appropriate for all patients has the potential for effecting significant changes in emotional disorder and for opening lives. This book was written for the wider dissemination of this knowledge.

About the Author

My interest in psychiatry was kindled at 16 years of age, the effect of a schoolboy argument. My opponent had declared, "You don't even know who Freud is." That led to Freud's Studies on Hysteria, which I comprehended only to the extent that I realized that the subject was fascinating.

Many years later I was preparing to enter psychoanalytic treatment and training. In a didactic course in psychoanalytic theory, I was not always satisfied by the analyst-instructor's answers to questions but assumed that that was the state of the art at the this time. As I came to know the training analysts, I was having difficulty finding one to whom I would entrust my psyche.

At this time a scholarly friend invited me to read a book he had just finished by Wilhelm Reich. I refused, with the explanation, "He's crazy." Challenged to support my claim, I could offer only that it was general knowledge; so I agreed to read the book.

By chance the book provided clear answers to some of the questions the teacher in the psychoanalytic course had fumbled. In succession I read all of Reich's books that were available and enjoyed a "Eureka!" experience (the modern equivalent is "Yeah!"). Later I discovered that this immediate feeling of rightness was common to colleagues who entered orgonomy.

It was evident that this was the therapy, and, if possible, the therapist I had sought. I applied for an interview with Reich in Forest Hills and was accepted as a patient, conditionally (as was his custom). He made it clear that I was simply a patient -- not a special case like a physician-patient or a trainee, or student.

Reich later moved to Maine and I followed for treatment and, later, training. So far as I am aware, I was his last trainee.

Morton Herskowitz, D.O., F.A.C.N.

Chapter 1
What is the cure? But first, what is the disease?

"I was feelin' very bad, scared of everything, even to go out of my house. No doctor was doin' nothin' for me except to make me very dopey. So a lady down the street told me about the gypsy man who was very good. So I went to see him, and he said he could get me better. He held an egg to my head here, and he said he was getting' the bad thoughts out. Then he made me swallow three eggs. I had to eat them raw. Then I started vomicking, and I tell you doctor I never vomicked like that in my whole life. Later on he brought in the pan and showed me what I vomicked-up. There was a mean little snake in there; that's what was makin' me feel so bad."

This tale told by a patient in a psychiatric clinic defines the therapeutic ideal -- to find the definitive cure for the comprehended disease, to administer the specific antibiotic with which to conquer the emotional infection. The gypsy man, alas, failed to duplicate his marvelous cure in a subsequent episode. Psychiatric theory was not enriched.

Psychiatry has no dearth of theories. Someone who took the trouble to count, listed more than two hundred psychotherapeutic regimens, each with its own theoretic base. Admittedly, some of these are variants on a basic theme, such as the slightly deviant schools of psychoanalysis. Even so, the number and diversity of approaches to the treatment of emotional disorder must be dismaying to the patient seeking treatment. Should the emotional tension with which he cannot cope be relieved with drugs, or by formal psychoanalysis? Or can he be trained out of his difficulty in a behavioral program in which he will learn new accommodations through rewards or punishments? Possibly, what he experiences as symptomatic simply requires a fresh weighing of what he values in life, with increased emphasis on spiritual accounting and de-emphasis of his personal pain.

Are his symptoms an inevitable consequence of being middle-aged and middle-class, or were they programmed in his genes? Will touching and communal nude bathing make him easier? Can he dance his anxiety out of his bones? Should someone act the role of father so that he may finally confront him? Or must he scream the pain of being born?

It is axiomatic in medicine that theories proliferate when the disease is not comprehended. Before the discovery of the specific organism and the specific antibiotic, infectious diseases were treated by such diverse means as exorcism or bloodletting; theories of what caused the disorder and what comprised the disease abounded. Once the cause is known and the process is understood, the multiplicity of theories ceases.

The problem of understanding and treating emotional disorders is multidimensional. It is clear that in some cases genetic endowment plays a role. It is equally apparent that social influences, especially in the earliest years, are instrumental in creating emotional disorder. Having observed that both nature and nurture play their part, what shall we consider the essence of the disturbance to be? Is it the troublesome symptom per se ? Or is it the inability to relate to other humans, which we can usually discern? Is there a chemical derangement at the root of all emotional disorder? We are aware that emotions are mediated chemically, that in some cases we can influence the course of disease by altering the chemical substrate. Is this the core of the matter -- the touchstone to effecting "cures"? What of insight? It is apparent that there are techniques which assist us in revealing how we are enthralled and how we become bound to our demons. Do we free ourselves in discovering the process? Each of these approaches has validity; yet we are left with a wonderment.

The behaviorist is clear in his mind -- the symptom is the disease. "You are afraid to walk over the bridge. I shall teach you to cross bridges and you will be well." Many years ago one of my patients was serving an internship under one of the foremost behavioral therapists. She came to her treatment session fresh from a conference in which her mentor had demonstrated the successful treatment of a phobic reaction in the patient. "He (the therapist) said the patient was cured," she exclaimed, "but I know the guy and he's an emotional wreck. He's a miserable, incompetent human being who's a wreck minus a phobia. That's cured?"

Patients on chemical treatment sometimes improve. The depressives may run a shorter course of depression on their drugs. On their lithium, the manic depressives may suffer fewer and less severe episodes of their illness and experience longer remissions. The schizophrenics may be relieved of their delusions and hallucinations with neuroleptic drugs, although they often purchase this relief at the price of the deadening of their spirit, living their lives in apathy. The neurotics gain symptomatic relief from their tranquilizers, as attested to by the fact that these are the most widely used drugs in the country. None of these drugs combats the disorder the way an antibiotic combats infection. Rather, they neutralize the symptoms, as insulin neutralizes the pancreatic deficiency in diabetes. Just as the successful use of insulin indicates the presence of diabetes, the use of the psychopharmacological drugs advertise: "Depression, schizophrenia, neurosis exist here."

Does insight into our feelings, actions, and symptoms liberate us from the process that creates them? On one hand we have evidence that it may. Many have experienced some relief from the combined processes of verbal ventilation and insight. Yet many others have not. I am reminded of a patient who came to me after eleven years of formal psychoanalysis. "I could write several volumes about what I learned about myself in analysis, but I've got the same damned symptoms I started with," he said. Freud was aware of this problem. He assumed that psychoanalysis was not successful when it proceeded as an exercise in cerebration. It was most effective when emotions were freed in tandem with insights. Unfortunately, there is no way that psychoanalysis can ensure that emotional depths will be uncovered in its exploration of the unconscious. Largely through the work of Wilhelm Reich, psychoanalysis increased its efficiency in this regard with the technique of analyzing the character structure. However, it is apparent that even character analysis is a roundabout way to repressed emotions.

The confusion about the proper method of treating emotional disorders is equaled by the disarray of concepts regarding the disease itself. Using schizophrenia as an example: on the most superficial level, what the American psychiatrist labels schizophrenia is not necessarily what the Russian psychiatrist calls schizophrenia; and the British psychiatrist might disagree with both. Some psychiatrists have made the case that schizophrenic patients within the asylum walls are less insane than their keepers and visitors. They say that compared to the patients, society is the madder. Obviously, the patient who complains that his neighbor is aiming a (nonexistent) x-ray machine at his genitals is suffering from delusional thinking. But what of the delusions we concede to one-another: I will allow that your Lord was born of a virginal conception if you allow that my God has forbidden me to eat shellfish and pig.

Most of us will agree on the worst cases. Clearly, the patient who sits in his catatonic trance mute, bone-still, with static eyes, is in the grip of an emotional malady. But let us consider two other cases. On the one hand is a woman patient who suffers from attacks of anxiety. Periodically she is troubled with a sense of oppression in her chest; her heart races; she feels suddenly cold and frightened. Though she is bright, sensitive, has warm relationships, enjoys her work, her symptoms label her a psychiatric patient. On the other hand is her dull, unfeeling, uninterested spouse. He moves through his life unrelated to the world outside his capsule. He has no symptoms, except he cannot fathom much more than mere existence. He will never by a psychiatric patient. Though he is symptom-free he is far more crippled emotionally, than she.

Symptoms, then, are not necessarily the truest index of emotional sickness. They are but one manifestation of disorder. Emotional disease may also proclaim its existence in such shortcomings as an inability to empathize or a failure to be moved deeply by nature or art. These feelings indicate a malfunction beyond specific symptoms and beyond particular aberrant behavior patterns. The source of the malfunction is the disordered character structure.

In his early work with character, Reich worked only with behavioral manifestations of character, investigating, for example, why the patient always agreed or always disagreed, why he came late to appointments, why she said everything with a smile. With focus and study he came to recognize that the flaws of character are written in the body. Dulled eyes, a tight jaw, a stiff neck, a tight throat, raised shoulders, held breath, taut loins, tight buttocks-- these were the physical, the biological statements of character disorder. He came to recognize that these areas of tension were the way human organisms repress emotions, and that this process altered the energy economy of the total organism. He called the process armoring. When armoring is reflected in attitudinal behavior, it is called character armoring; when it is manifested in bodily tension it is called muscular armoring.

Except in those instances when it results from toxins and physical deformity such as brain tumors, armoring is the substrate of emotional (mental) disorder. Armoring is where body and mind touch to effect abnormal behavior. Conversely, the unarmored organism is not beset with distortion as it reacts to environmental stimuli. It feels pain when hurt, moves with joy and thrill when that is possible, senses the longing of knowing and reaching out to the natural world. It is sentient and is freely mobile. It has bounce.

The concept of armoring does not exclude discoveries of the psychopharmacological researchers. It is clear that armoring affects hormones and enzymes. The mind and the flesh and the chemical substrates are of one piece. Anxiety and epinephrine are inseparable, just as stubbornness and stiff necks are.

To return to our original inquiry: The disease is not the symptom which the patient perceives or the behavior which his associates observe. These are the demonstrable effects of an underlying disorder of character, the result of physical armoring. The symptoms and the behavior may be altered by various means -- chemical, physical, psychological, but the underlying disorder persists which ordains that the life will be lived with constraint. There will be limitations on feeling, thinking, acting, relating; and these limitations will set a qualitative stamp on that life. We gird ourselves against our terrors by armoring, and the girders become a strait jacket on our lives.

Emotional dysfunction extends beyond symptoms and behavioral deviations; it encompasses our limitations in reacting wholly to our world. Armored humans suffer from a defect in metabolizing life.

As we live our lives of "quiet desperation," we are, for the most part, not aware of how we are bound. We demonstrate for freedom of speech unmindful of how we constrain ourselves to think only within narrow paths. We are so fearful of floating in the mystery of existence that we rush to calm our anxiety with the ready-made answers of organized religion or put on a brave show with scientific formulas which we have inherited. We rationalize our fear of fighting when we are angered. We stiffen when we are in danger of feeling tenderness. We fuck when we are in peril of loving.

Wilhelm Reich discovered the process of armoring and its meaning in our lives. He also devised the technique with which we could attempt to dissolve the armoring -- a method he called psychiatric orgone therapy. It was the first therapy which recognized the significance of armoring in psychiatric disorders.

Psychiatric orgone therapy is not a cure-all. It is a painstaking system of therapy which entails some degree of physical and often a great deal of emotional discomfort. It has succeeded in effecting rewarding changes in the lives of many patients.

Chapter 2
The First Session: Observation

The point of the initial contact with the patient is to evaluate his character structure. The therapist first observes the patient's behavior, which will reveal the character armoring; then as the patient lies on the couch, the therapist observes the places where the body tenses, which reveal physical armoring. This evaluation enables the therapist first to establish whether the patient is a suitable candidate for therapy and then to draw up an initial plan of operation.

As used here, the term "first session" includes the procedure from the time the patient enters the office through the initial biophysical evaluation as he lies on the couch. In real time, the observation on the couch may not occur on the initial visit, sometimes not for months.

The therapist has an impression of the patient before any words are uttered. The gait, dress, facial expressions and attitude all speak of the particular way this individual moves through life. The therapist encourages the patient to talk about the complaints and symptoms that brought him into therapy. Sometimes a brief history will suffice, and in that case the patient may be observed on the couch in the initial visit to determine the extent of the physical armoring and to begin to relieve it. One would then leave the more complete history-taking for a later time. This would be the likely procedure when the patient's complaint and suffering are acute, and relief is a more important, immediate goal than a full history. In other cases, one might spend the first three or four visits listening to the patient's story, eliciting a detailed psychiatric and medical history, all the while evaluating his behavioral characteristics. During this period, the therapist may determine that the patient is not a good candidate for psychiatric orgone therapy because his motivation is poor or the character is brittle and could not tolerate assault. In this case the therapist might refer the patient to a conventional psychiatrist who could as competently give the patient emotional support or help to manipulate the environment without threatening the character structure.

In some cases the therapist decides that, given a certain history and character, it would be judicious simply to talk with the patient for weeks or months until the patient has gained sufficient confidence to begin the physical work on the couch.

Regarding motivation: some patients come to therapy only to satisfy their wife's (husband's) request, determined not to do the necessary work. They are sent back home. Others may come to psychiatric orgone therapy because they regard it as anti-establishment (which it is, but not in their political sense), and because its the "hip" therapy. Whether the therapist chooses to treat these patients depends on the character structure behind the attitude. In some cases these attitudes would be superficial and might yield to therapeutic pressures. In others they might represent negativism of such huge proportions as to stand fixedly opposed to a therapeutic approach. A sensible therapist would send such patients packing.

There is an implicit agreement with every patient who comes to therapy: both the patient and the therapist are free to terminate treatment when either is dissatisfied with the course and progress of the therapy. The patient may not understand well enough that severe dislocations, both personal and social, occur as he progresses in therapy. As this becomes increasingly clear, he may become frightened and choose to withdraw. This is his right.

A strictly observing Catholic young man came to therapy with moderately severe emotional symptomatology. I was impressed with his seriousness. Both he and I put a great deal of energy into the first sessions, and things were moving well. He came to the fourth session and requested that we talk, rather than work on the couch. He asked whether continuing in therapy might alter his religious beliefs. "It all depends on how far we get," I answered. "A certain amount of loosening can be accomplished without affecting them. But when we get beyond a certain depth, they will undoubtedly come into question." "In that case," he said, "I think I'd rather not come any more."

He returned after six months. "If my religion is valid, it will stand up against any rational thing that happens," he reasoned, "and it not, then I'd better find out now. So let's start again."

The therapist may discover as the therapy progresses that the patient has arrived at a point of equilibrium where the intensity of the symptoms has decreased and the armoring is looser, but still present. He may decide that to continue beyond this juncture would expose the patient to emotional vicissitudes beyond his tolerance, and he may propose that therapy be terminated at that point, at least temporarily. Or the therapist may become disenchanted with hopes for further progress by repeated evidence of the patient's failure to cooperate, by continuing to indulge his appetite for drugs, for example, and he may discontinue the therapy.

In psychiatric orgone therapy the patient is observed from two aspects. First, the therapist gains insight into the patient's psychological side through the symptoms, the historical survey, the observed behavior. Then, to complete his picture, the physician must also learn how and where emotional repression is represented in the physical structure -- where the body is armored.

In the treatment room the patient is requested to take off his clothes and to lie on the couch. The general rule in therapy is that patients of the opposite sex are treated in their underclothes, and patients of the same sex may be treated in the nude or in underclothes, as the therapist sees fit. The patient removes his clothing because the therapist is constantly observing bodily changes: skin color, skin temperature, hair erection (gooseflesh), nipple erection, the visual and palpatory signs of muscular tension. Another benefit of the clothing removal is that to some extent clothing is used as a social armor and its removal renders the patient more revealed; there is one less place to hide. There are, however, no rigid rules. Patients who are embarrassed to take off their clothes might be treated clothed for a number of sessions until they feel more comfortable disrobing.

The fact that patients undress for therapy has, of course, occasioned sick fantasies in some minds. *Honi soit qui mal y pense.*

To prepare himself for theoretical discussions that will follow, the reader might imagine himself sitting beside the therapist to see what he sees as he observes the patient on the couch in his first session. The thoughtful and observant visitor may be surprised at some of the reactions he witnesses, and his interest in the theory might be enlivened by his curiosity.

Before the therapist proceeds, he observes the patient before him. Is he at relative ease, or is he upset? Does he lie prone, supine, in a fetal position? Are his legs crossed, spread open, separated with toes turned in, or bent at the knees? Is he pale, hands sweaty and cold, pupils dilated? Is his face masked, serious, sad, embarrassed, expectant? Does it look as if it will break into a smile? Are there any sharp lines of color demarcation (florid face and neck, pale chest, for example), any sharp lines of temperature change (warm abdomen, cold loins)? What body areas are held in tension, which parts relaxed? This initial reading often reveals more than a patient could say in hours.

Patient #1

A middle-aged male is lying staring at the ceiling. His legs are crossed, hands clasped resting on his abdomen. He is literally holding himself together. Palms are cool, slightly moist. Occasionally he sneaks a furtive sidelong glance at me, then returns to the ceiling. His chest barely moves; breathing is revealed mostly by abdominal excursions. The jaw is held rigidly and the lips are tightly pressed.

I instruct him to breathe with his chest, raising his chest with a full inspiration and permitting the chest to collapse with a long, full expiration. I demonstrate the breathing. The patient begins to breathe, but as he continues he begins to catch his breath in his throat at the height of inspiration. This is corrected with some difficulty. The patient is now staring more fixedly at the ceiling, and he is clenching his jaw more tightly. Now his palms are quite cold, betraying his anxiety. As he continues he asks, "What shall I do now?" He is advised to continue doing what he's doing. After a while an involuntary laugh breaks through, which he attempts to suppress. "Let it go," I say, "let whatever happens, happen." Despite this instruction, he continues to deny the laughter, but after a while it breaks through more strongly and is more difficult to hold back. I pry his jaws open and instruct him to keep his mouth open and to increase the volume of the sound. Now the laughter changes to guffawing and the patient is rocking with it. "What the hell am I laughing about? There's nothing funny," he manages to say as he continues to be seized with his laughter, tears now falling down his cheeks. At times he manages to quiet the laughter and he continues to breathe, and then it explodes again. "This is crazy," he keeps repeating as he laughs.

Gradually the frequency and intensity of the laughter subsides until he is only breathing. His chest moves more easily now and there is a satisfaction in his breathing. "Can I stop now?" he asks, and I agree. He dresses and as he leaves he says, "That was wild, I feel a little nervous, but I feel good."

Patient #2

An attractive young woman in her thirties lies on the couch in apparent bewilderment. "Are you Dr. A. (her referring physician)?" she asks. "No," I answer, "I am Dr. H.; Dr. A sent you to me." "I think I like him better than you," she comments, looking at the corners of the room in an attempt to orient herself. "Are you going to hurt me or do anything bad to me?" she wonders aloud, and I assure her that I am not. "Would you open your mouth," she asks, and when I do she carefully examines the oral cavity and its contents for several minutes. "Okay," she says, and she gently shuts my mouth.

As I inspect and feel her body there is no place that is tightly held, except for slight tension in the cervical area and the scalp. She barely moves her chest when she breathes. The major pathology is in her face. Her eyes are set dully in her head, almost stupidly, though it is clear that she is quite intelligent. Her extremities are warm; no anxiety present. From time to time she pokes at her ear and grimaces as if to push her eyes forward in her sockets.

When asked to breathe, her chest moves fairly freely, not in a full and deep respiratory excursion, but not tightly bound, either. However, she can only take four or five successive breaths, then her breathing diminishes to its former quiescent state. Repeatedly she is urged to try to keep the breathing going, but it is apparently more than she can do. "Can we try something else?" she asks. Admonishing her to continue to breathe steadily, I move a small flashlight back and forth in front of her face, then in haphazard directions before her eyes, instructing her to follow the light by moving her eyes only, holding her head still. She can do this for only short periods, then her eyes cross or she looks away and goes blank. She is clearly unhappy with her performance, and at each new attempt she seems determined to continue longer .

Now I ask her to hold her head in place and to move her eyes from wall to wall around the room in a large circle. I ask her to do this as quickly as possible, and not merely to move her eyes but to see as much as possible as they move. As she performs this task, her eyes stick in the upraised position. She has difficulty moving them to see the wall behind her. Instead of moving in successive, equally spaced circles, her eyes make a single loop and become stuck at the top. We work on the movement at the top of the circle; she is becoming frustrated and her lips and mouth are forming into a pouty little girl cry, which soon erupts. We return to the eye movement for a little while, then to simply breathing. She reaches for my hand and holds it as she continues. I announce the end of the session, and she says, "That was good."

Patient #3

A seven-year-old boy is lying apprehensively on the couch. His pupils are wide. He's staring off to the side but watching me out of the corner of his eye. His chest feels solid as a wooden cage. I have never felt such a chest in a child, only rarely in an adult and then only in elderly patients, suffering from pulmonary disorders, such as emphysema. The chest is held in a fixed inspiratory position. This patient has come not because of any respiratory problem but because of a behavior disorder. He is uncontrollable in school; and though he never causes serious trouble, he is constantly disruptive. The situation is similar at home. His mother says that though he's not really a bad boy, he wears her out with his constant minor transgression and excessive activity. The only symptom that is obviously related to his rigid-box chest is that of stuttering.

When he is asked to breathe, his chest remains immobile and his belly balloons up and down. I restrain the abdominal movement with one hand and press on his chest cautiously with each expiration (cautiously, because this chest is so brittle that I am wary of cracking a rib -- this in a seven-year old!). Nothing much is happening; there is still very little give in the chest.

I dig my fingers into his intercostal muscles (the muscles between the ribs) and he winces and squirms but doesn't utter a sound. "Doesn't it hurt?" I ask, and he nods that it does. "Then why don't you yell?" I say. He shrugs. "Come on now, yell," and I dig my fingers into his intercostals again. He grimaces, part jocular, part silly, part frightened, and utters the merest sound. He is squirming so that I have a battle to hold him in place with the unrelenting fingers digging into his chest. This continues until my fingers are aching. A few tears drop down his cheeks, but still no sound. All the while now his eyes are on me, and they are good eyes, looking me in the eye, sad. Partly because of my aching fingers and partly because I do not want to hurt him any more, I withdraw my hand. He takes one deep breath; his chest moves a little now.

Patient #4

A young lady in late adolescence, acutely anxious, is lying on the couch. She complains of difficulty in breathing and a feeling of constriction in her throat. She fidgets the sheet with the fingers of one hand and fingers her hair with the other; her feet and toes are in constant motion.

She is asked to breathe and has difficulty both in drawing a full breath and in letting the breath expire freely. As she continues to breathe, she becomes aware of tingling in her finger tips and this increases her fear. As the tingling proceeds into her hands, she cries, "Stop it, please!" She is instructed now to punch the couch and yell simultaneously. She punches tentatively at first, then with more vigor. Her voice moves from innocuous sound to the beginning of a yell, but before it can proceed to a full yell it turns into a whine. I press hard on muscles in her neck, which have become tense bands since she first attempted to yell. She voices the pain briefly, then bursts into sobs, which continue for the duration of the session.

Patient #5

A grossly obese young man in his twenties lies on the couch, and one has the impression that the most significant thing going on is that he is glad to get the load of his feet.

In response to the request to breathe, he appears to cooperate. The chest is moderately mobile. The neck is somewhat stiff and the eyes are vacuous. When asked to look at me as he breathes, he follows orders and looks at me with the same blank eyes that formerly stared into space. When asked to follow a light, his eyes move with momentary ambition, then dull out again. An attempt to provoke his neck musculature by prodding leaves me wondering whether I am causing him any pain through all that fat. He continues to breathe dutifully. Nothing happens. I ponder how, and whether, I can get to him at all through his glassed eyes and fortress of lard.

Patient #6

A quiet, tight-lipped man in his forties, taut-necked, chest-held, staring-off, lies on the couch, breathing. As he breathes, his shoulders become more rigid. I poke between his shoulder blades and he says, "Ouch! Don't do that," with a smile. I continue poking, but harder. The smile becomes continuous and he keeps murmuring, "No, don't do that." I encourage him to punch the couch and he counters with "I'm not angry at the couch," smiling. Imitating his words and vapid smile, I urge him to hit the couch, all the while digging into his shoulder. He hits the couch innocuously with open hands; I urge him to close his fists and punch with all his might. Gradually he increases the pitch of his punching until he is emotionally involved. Now he is really punching and yelling, "Damn you!" He breaks out into a body-wide cold sweat and I tell him to stop. Now his chest is moving freely, spontaneously. His hands are ice cold. I tell him to quiet his breathing down a little, and he becomes a little warmer. I ask to whom he was yelling "Damn you!" and he says he doesn't know. The session ends with the chest still free; he wears an almost beatific expression. His outstretched hands have a gross tremor and his heart still races. He is advised to rest in the waiting room till the tremor disappears.

Patient #7

A patient in her mid-twenties lies breathing and continually interrupts herself to ask whether she's doing it correctly. With a little impatience, I direct her to shut-up and resume breathing. Now, rather than vocally request confirmation of her performance, her eyes seek out mine and they keep asking, "Is this all right?"

I explain that she is not supposed to gain my approval but to fathom and express the hidden parts of herself. She starts again with deeper sighs, now tinged with the breath of emotion. Her eyes become less guarded, softer. She is permitting herself to sink into the quiet lake of her own feelings. In a mini-second she rouses her eyes toward mine and asks, "Is that better?" Caught between the impulse to break into laughter and the desire to throttle her, I begin to explain her resistance. The session ends on this exposition.

Chapter 3
The Concept of Armoring

The reader acquainted only with conventional psychotherapeutic techniques will have noted that there is scant resemblance between the modalities he knows and the events reported in the preceding chapter. The verbal communication that is the hallmark of the dynamic psychotherapies is almost nonexistent in the reported sessions (though therapy includes times of talking). A patient unsophisticated in psychiatric practice once reported to me in amusement that his friend was seeing a psychiatrist, "and all they did was talk."

What is the reader to make of the phenomena witnessed in those first sessions? The first patient was made to breathe more fully than usual. The breath caught in his throat, and when that was corrected, he inexplicably was seized with uncontrollable laughter.

The second patient, disoriented and disorganized, achieved some temporary clarity and satisfaction by the hour's end -- from eye exercises? From the brief spell of crying?

The seven-year-old boy had little reaction to the prodding and poking, though his chest at the end of the session was slightly more flexible. But where is the connection between his behavior disorder and the fact that his chest was rigid and became a little looser in his session?

The key that opens the door to our comprehension of the data is the process that Reich, with fine reason, called armoring. Armoring is both a physiological and psychological condition. It represents the physiological anchoring of emotional repression. Emotional repression implies an opposition of forces: buried emotions struggle up toward expression and are pushed down toward repression. In this process of constant opposition, energy is continuously consumed. With armoring, energy is constantly withdrawn from the organism's free use and spent in the ceaseless battle to bury emotions.

Though Reich discovered the meaning of armoring for science, men have always known of armoring and reacted to it. The great novelists have observed it clearly when they described character. The frozen curl of the lips and the dilated nostrils presaged weeping, the catch in the breath when something that was about to be expressed must suddenly be concealed. Whatever the covert expression, artists have read and correctly translated it. Our response to these literary descriptions shows that we, too, know. Perhaps we need to be reminded with verbal pointers before our consciousness is jolted into recognition, but the awareness is there.

To some extent each of us governs our interpersonal responses by reading the other's armoring. We say of stiff-necked persons that they are unyielding. We are wary of the biting anger in a person with clenched jaws. We despair of being understood by one with dulled eyes.

Our own armoring determines how we will respond to the armoring of another person. It is obvious that the distracted eyes not only bump into furniture and trip over their own feet; they do not "see" people either. If your chest is tight, you are unaware that most chests are held; whereas when my chest is free, I experience the tension in your chest empathically as a tendency to constrict my own chest. When I am with another who is "loose-chested," I can breathe more freely. We may dislike in others armoring that we ourselves have. For example, if I am even dimly aware of the spite expressed in my lips, and it's an annoyance to me, when I read (albeit unconsciously) the spite in your mouth, it may be the cause of instant antipathy towards you, though I know nothing else about you. To the extent to which we are so accustomed to our armoring that we are dead to it, we are not aware of it in others. Insofar as we are free of particular armoring, we can read it clearly in others.

The problem of armoring pertains not only to physical and emotional health, but to insight, perspective, world-view. Through history the unarmored human has suffered from the armoring of his peers. To his clear insight they have replied, "But I have eyes and I don't see that!" "I never felt that in my vagina," say the armored pelves. Until now we have failed to distinguish between organisms that function freely and naturally and those that function in a distorted fashion. We call them all "organisms" and ascribe equal powers to them. To have failed to apply the modifier "armored" has tumbled us into a semantic error of the highest order and led us into a world of confusion.

Reich's contribution is not merely that he calls our attention to the armoring process, but that he describes the resulting drain of the organism's energy. The difference between observing and truly perceiving an event in its proper scientific perspective is enormous. For millennia we displaced water in our tubs and watched apples falling from trees but learned nothing about our universe.

Reich reveals to us that wherever there is emotional repression there is a concomitant protoplasmic contraction in the body. Because this physical tension tends to become chronic with time, binds energy and constricts the free pulsation of our bodies, it is truly an armor that imprisons us for life. Our physical armoring characterizes our body just as our characterologic armoring delineates our behavior. Armoring is the point at which biology meets psychology, or (another way of saying the same thing) armoring is the physiological anchoring of the aberrant behavior. The elucidation of this concept has given us a rock upon which we can stand to evaluate human events and see man in relation to his universe. It is the means by which we can determine where man deviates from his nature. There has never been a discovery of greater human import.

If we are all armored -- and we are -- then the history of humanity has been the history of an emotionally and physically crippled animal. Our revolutions and our religions fail to liberate us because after we have struggled to free ourselves, we still find ourselves within the same cocoon that we continuously weave. Armored man creates institutions which, on the one hand, promise to free him from his tension ("Love God and you will be saved."), and on the other, deliver him right back to armoring in perpetuity. For the truth is that like the long-termer who has been imprisoned from youth, we have made some peace with our prison; and though we hope for it, we harbor a deep fear against the day of release when we will be discharged into the open, unknown, sunlit world outside. This fear conditions every gesture, every act, every opinion.

An old-fashioned cartoonist might portray Aspiring Humanity as a soaring creature beating his wings so rapidly that he creates the illusion of flying. All the while the soarer's feet are clasped in the maw of a mythic beast with sly eyes -- Human Armoring.

Once aware of the armoring process, we are amazed that we failed to discern it before. A young mother now notes that each time the family visits her in-laws, her infant son returns with a rigid back and unease that requires weeks of soft eye-contact to dissipate. She never saw it before; she only knew that the visits affected his eating pattern. The ease with which armoring can be acquired is most obvious in young children (though the rapidity with which adults can develop headaches in uncomfortable situations leaves them not far behind). A patient describing the rigid neck and shoulders and the cold extremities of a three-month old relative said, "He's well-developed beyond his age, both physiologically and neurotically."

To graphically portray the effect of armoring, let us think of a freely pulsating bladder -- a jellyfish, say, and watch for a while as it glides gracefully from its expansive to its contractile phase, and back. In this pulsating dance there is beauty, ease, a rightness that is duplicated throughout unarmored nature -- in the lope of a bear, the reaching-out and arriving of the amoeba, the peristalsis of the mammalian intestine, the contraction and expansion of the heart, the wave of a sidewinder snake. (Says armored man: "That snake motion gives me the willies; the jellyfish too, and the beating heart, for that matter.)

To demonstrate the effect of armoring, let us place a rubber band across the jellyfish's middle. Where the jellyfish once pulsated as a single unit, expanding and contracting freely, the rubber band causes the jellyfish to expand and contract in disconnected segments. The beauty of the pulsation is gone. The animal functions as much in response to the constricting rubber band as it once did to the great ocean in which it lived. It is cut off from direct contact with its cosmos; instead of being beautiful, it is now unnatural. The band has not only interfered with the physical aspect of pulsation; it has, in effect, made the jellyfish into a different creature, and affected all of its functions.

Armoring distorts human functioning to the same extent that the rubber band deformed the jellyfish. Innocent impulses become cockeyed impulses. Armoring transmutes an organism born to religious awe (cosmic longing) into one who calls circumcision of newborns and celibacy a religious duty. It changes eyes that linger and look deeply, as a young child's, into eyes that look sidelong and turn away. Aggression, which is the instrument for overcoming obstacles and leads us to explore, becomes the tool of hatred and money acquisitiveness. Our bodies lose their ease and grace and become stiff, wheezy, dyspeptic and constipated. Our armoring disfigures us literally and spiritually.

If we return to the example of the jellyfish and the rubber band, we can illustrate other aspects of the armoring process. If there were only one band and it was not too constricting, the organism might almost function as a jellyfish, albeit distracted and uncomfortable. But if there were many bands dividing the entire jellyfish circle into segments, or if there were one broad, taut band constricting the animal almost in two, functioning would be grossly distorted to the point that all the organism's energies would be used in merely surviving. This condition is the case of a large part of humanity. Whereas the lightly or more discreetly armored humans can pursue their work and expend energies for good or evil, the large number of heavily armored people have ceased to struggle, they wear out their days in unfeeling existence. These, not the disturbed psychotic or the complaining neurotic, are the sickest humans.

For academic purposes, armoring can be viewed from either the psychological or somatic side. Thus, we take one of these inert humans and, by skewing our vision, view him purely psychologically. He lives a life of dull routine. He works mechanically at a dull job. He comes home and drinks one or two quarts of beer, eats, watches TV and often falls asleep engaged in this activity. He has sexual intercourse with his wife on Saturdays and holidays, stops at the tap room to drink beer with the guys on Fridays and usually gets home a little drunk. He has a big breakfast on Sundays and spends most of the day supine watching TV. He goes for a two-week vacation at the same rooming house at the shore each year. His children visit every few months; once he has inquired as to their health and jobs, he has little to say. He is probably roused most by a good game on TV. He says that he is not prejudiced, but he has some feeling about the blacks who are beginning to move into his neighborhood, thinking of property values and the principle that "people should stay with their own." Nothing in the world moves him very much, positively or negatively, but he says, "I'm not complaining." He hates fights and gets along "ok" with the guys. "They don't bother me and I don't bother them." In fact, his life was satisfactory to him until he sustained a minor injury at work and became increasingly apprehensive of working at his machine. He arrived at the point where he fears going to work and concocts transparent excuses to stay at home. The fact that an injury touches some deep anxiety raises him above the most lifeless of the inert. Another might have had an arm severed and gone on dully.

What does the physical armoring look like on this level? His eyes are lifeless and never make contact. His face is a mask of blandness, lined only by age and not by character. The muscles of his neck are flabby, lacking tonicity. No gag reflex is elicited when he inserts his fingers deep into his throat. His chest barely moves with respiration; no matter how he tries to breathe deeply, he cannot move his chest. His abdomen is hard. His pelvis is dead. The picture is the same from the behavioral and physical sides. He is barely alive, though he may continue to exist for many years.

The functional identity of the character (psychological) and muscular (somatic) armoring can also be revealed in examination. To attack either exposes the patient to the anxiety that armoring holds in abeyance. A patient whose intolerance of hostility is hidden behind a facade of passivity and submissiveness can be provoked verbally by an insulting description of his spineless behavior. If the provocation is sufficiently skillful, the patient will react with anger. As he does, his anxiety will be revealed in his cold sweaty hands and tachycardia (increased heart beat rate). Or the same patient, who, when asked to punch the couch with anger, always flailed weakly and without affect, now, with painful prodding of his shoulder armoring, begins to really punch, muttering, "Damn you, damn you." A cold sweat suffuses the entire body surface, the pupils are wide, the patient is in fear of his own hostility.

The armoring, characterologic or muscular, allays anxiety. In the performance of this function, it establishes a somewhat peaceful equilibrium for the organism at the expense of full contact with the environment and with its own core. In the example just cited, the patient could neither perceive his own hostility nor express it appropriately in the world. He lost the freedom of spontaneous reaction and the fullness of his emotional capacity for quietude. He traded true and lively communication for a predictable, boring "niceness" which characterized him. In place of free and genuine contact, he exhibited a substitute contact, a social facade behind which the reality of his person was diminished. He no longer pulsated along with the jellyfish and the amoeba.

A skilled observer can predict that there will be little or no emotional reaction from an individual with strongly armored eyes and rigidly held chest who is suddenly bereft of a loved one. At most there will be annoyance or discomfiture at the sudden change in his living arrangements. In fact, the problem as stated is inaccurate, because our armored example is incapable of possessing a "loved" one. The unarmored individual faced with the same circumstance may react in a variety of ways. He may withdraw into solitude so he can concentrate on his pain, not distracted by well-wishers; he may sob for hours or days; he may think deeply on life and death; he may seek out other intimates so that they can communicate the depth of their feelings. The only element of <u>his</u> behavior that is predictable is that the experience of death will move him deeply. The particular way that he will react is totally unpredictable. The difference between unarmored and armored behavior is the difference between a variable curve and a straight line.

Armoring, to the extent that it is a temporarily useful function, tends to perpetuate itself. The infant who first discovers that by holding its breath it can momentarily decrease the intensity of the huge emotional pain it is feeling will tend to hold its breath when it experiences its next lesser pain. If this process is not corrected, it will have an armored chest by early childhood with which it can diminish the experience of all pain. The armored child, now adult, will conduct his life to avoid any exposure to pain, maintaining the integrity of his armoring and, unfortunately, grossly limiting his exposure to life's experience. When he is a parent, he will be closed to his child's pain. The child, lacking parental sustenance in painful situations, will soon learn to armor in turn. Thus and thus, for generations.

The question, "Where did armoring begin?" is an interesting one. From his history we know that man, at least Western man, has been armored for millennia. We know that there are variations in the intensity of armoring within a culture and between cultures. Some primitive peoples are relatively unarmored in comparison to us, for example, the Trobrianders as described by Malinowski, or the Maasai in Kenya. Other primitives, the Melanesian Dobuans, for example, are, judging by their behavior, far more armored than we; among the Dobu, treachery and hostility are social virtues. The degree to which society has advanced materially is therefore no criterion of the extent of armoring within that society. Why are humans, so far as we can tell, and excepting our domesticated animals, the only armored mammals? (I refer only to mammals because we do not understand the behavior of extra-mammalian animals enough to evaluate it.)

In his book Cosmic Superimposition, Reich tackles the problem of the origin of armoring. In what he calls "more than empty speculation" but " less than practicable theory," he postulates that at a point in the dim past when man became capable of reasoning <u>beyond</u> the immediate circumstance in which he found himself (i.e. reasoning not merely to discover the best way to extricate himself from a dangerous situation or how to accomplish a work task), when reasoning became a

Ding an sich -- he knew that he knew -- the perception was so frightening that he armored against this inner fright, and the process has continued in the species. The consonance of this postulate with the biblical loss of Eden for having tasted of the fruit of the tree of knowledge is fascinating, making allowance for a literal translation of knowledge as knowledge vs. the biblical implication of "knowledge" as sexuality.

This postulate, poses difficulties as we apply it to our own experience. In relatively unarmored children, as their perceptions deepen and their awareness increases, chronic armoring does not attend the process. Their armoring correlates with observable social traumata. This, of course, does not invalidate Reich's hypothesis, because the case of primitive man does not equal that of a growing modern child; it merely fails to add evidence. The definitive answer to this intriguing question is simply not known at this time.

Individual armoring is the thread from which the fabric of our society is woven. And on the other hand, society determines by which threads we shall pattern our lives. The relationship is reciprocally reinforcing. This relationship is the bottom reason why significant social change creeps at a wounded snail's pace. The "sins" that the biblical prophets railed against are still with us, undiminished. The religious institutions, designed to save our souls, are as blind and corrupt as when Jesus preached against them. Reich, in The Murder of Christ, refers to the relationship between man's armoring and the societal institutions which reinforce that armoring as "The Trap." Armored men, he believes, have always perceived their entrapment, if only dimly. They have murmured or shouted against it. Reformers have launched revolutions which were to free men from the trap. In the course of time each revolution failed; after a flurry of apparent freedom, men remained stuck where they had been. Curiously, those who pointed a way out of the trap were usually vilified and often persecuted.

There is a mean irony in man's attempt to escape the effects of his character. In their attempts to overcome prejudice, avarice, "sin", the reformer and the revolutionary palpitate for a moment in a wave of nobility and largesse. Then, when the reform or revolution achieves power, the position of the revolutionary party gradually hardens and develops its own prejudice, avarice, and "sin." Which evokes the next revolutionary.

Reich refers to the failure of leaders and seers to factor human armoring into their plan for a better world as a "biological miscalculation in the struggle for human freedom." The simple fact, Reich suggests, is that while men aspire to freedom, dignity, independence, joy, they are structurally incapable of achieving it. Freedom in the minds of the masses of humanity implies merely escape from under the oppressor's knuckles, which is reasonable enough, but insufficient. Once escaped, people must be capable of managing their lives rationally; they must have a scale of values that gives priority to the satisfaction of their deepest needs. Armored persons are so cut off from their own depth that they are not even aware of their deepest needs; and if they are "freed," they become lost in superficialities and excesses. They are so accustomed to direction from above that, given their own head, they are incapable of conducting their lives responsibly. Soon they cry for a new leader to whom they can entrust the course of their lives. So long as the human masses are armored, their social organization must reflect this biological distortion, and freedom is a chimera.

The condition of being a man in The Trap is frustrating. So many of us lead dull, unsatisfying, painful lives. We distract ourselves with entertainment, which wears thin. We keep busy to keep from feeling our emptiness. We champion causes, perhaps achieve a minor victory, and in time discover that we have not done much to fill our inner emptiness. Some of us find surcease through our guru, or Jesus. We put our hand in the palm of the Master and permit ourselves to be conducted through life -- cut-off somewhere, but guarded and peaceful. Others of us confine our lives to our work or champion causes to distract us from ourselves.

We are so blind to the fact that our entrapment is unnatural that an eminent American psychiatrist, Jules Masserman in The Practice of Dynamic Psychiatry proposes that we can live our lives only with a basic store of delusion.

„What in the world are delusions? and when in the name of heaven are they necessary? Let us now answer both tentatively, as follows: Delusions are the denials and the substitutive or compensatory beliefs necessary to make each man's world seem a little more like the heaven he so ardently desires. We dare not, then, disregard the psychological truism that such beliefs, in a truly humanitarian sense, are indeed sacred, and that we tamper with them at our patient's --and our own -- peril. Let us keep this theme implicit in all our discussions of psychotherapeutic techniques in the chapters that follow".

We make our way through the centuries leading "lives of quiet desperation" suspended on cords of delusion.

The critical question, then, is whether the character of modern man and his society flows from man's essential nature and is, in a deep sense, unalterable; or whether homo normalis and his institutions are the product of biological distortion. Those therapists who advocate that a patient "adjust" to his environment are obviously commenting on the essential "correctness" of things as they are, though they may simultaneously despair of the situation. Reich is the first to talk of society as the patient. To him homo normalis and the society that evolved from his structure are both deformed. This is certainly not to say that Reich is iconoclastic or cynical. Just as there are impulses toward health in the sickest patient, so are there wholesome tendencies in society. As illness is an attempt to right the pathology that affects the individual, the societal eruptions often reflect the same tendency. Whatever exists, Reich cautions, has its own good reason. We may recognize that the institution of organized religion causes a great deal of damage, that the institutional police can be repressive and brutal. But without the restraint of religion, men's sick sexuality would have freer play in the world (the fact that the religion also helped to create the sick sexuality does not bear on this argument immediately). Without the police force, the incidence of criminal activity would multiply wildly. The institutions reflect the societal sickness but are also the attempt to deal with it. To recognize the first property and disregard the second, and on this basis to call for the abolition of the institution would be socially irresponsible and would lead to chaos. Summary decapitation of social evils is a method that befits only the queen of hearts in Wonderland.

Some Properties of Armoring

A five-year-old boy lies in his bathtub enjoying the sensation of the warm water running over his skin, stroking his penis gently, immersed in the delicious sensation as his organ grows. Suddenly he is shocked by his mother and grandmother, who must have been standing at the open door. They rush in with ugly faces and shattering voices accusing him of heinous behavior, threatening to throw him out of the house if they ever catch him doing that again. He is utterly paralyzed.

His body feels sick -- numb, except that there is an aching pain in his penis. In that instant he thinks that he may die.

A patient in his mid-thirties is lying on the couch breathing freely, relaxed except for some minor finger movement. I have noted for some time that in anxious moments the patient's hands wander down to cover his penis and protect it. As I observe the patient in his quietly pleasurable breathing, I suddenly lunge toward the patient's genital region with a shout. (I dare to do this because, having known the patient for many months in therapy, I know that the patient is relatively unarmored down to his abdomen and pelvis.) The patient defends himself with an instantaneous rush of his hands to cover his genitals; his mouth and eyes fly open; pupils dilate; his skin blanches and he is frozen. The frozen attitude gradually shifts to one of deep belly sobs. When the sobbing subsides, he tells of the memory of the episode in the tub at age five -- a memory that had been repressed to this time.

The recovery of memories of acute emotional traumata is fairly common in the process of attacking armored segments. The memory is in the muscles.

An ambulatory schizophrenic patient in her mid-twenties lies on the couch following a flashlight with her eyes, which I move in quick, darting motions before her. We have worked intermittently for several years on freeing her armored eyes. We both recognize that she sees more now than ever before, that her eyes move more freely and that she can tolerate some limited expression of emotion in her eyes. At this point therapist and patient both assume that the regular trips in and out of institutions, which have persisted since pre-puberty, are a thing of the past. Mother says she is delighted with the progress.

Mother is a short, chubby, twittery walking Hallmark card. It is impossible to communicate with her on any meaningful level. As a therapist, I am completely sympathetic to the plight of the daughter of such an apparently pleasant, concerned, empty woman. The wonder is that the patient is still able to hear after all that twittering.

In all of the hard work on mobilizing the patient's deadened eyes, no repressed memories of situations with Mother, have been recovered. The reason is that Mother is not an acute trauma, though she completely immobilized her daughter's eyes. Mother is the insidious way things happened; she is a process. Mother leaves armoring without memory.

A sensitive and lively child is attacked repeatedly by an older and bigger boy at school. The child initially makes an attempt to fight back physically and is beaten badly. Next, he makes an attempt to verbally assault his oppressor and is beaten again. He finally discovers that he can use his superior wit to make sly, derogatory remarks that go above the head of his tormentor. Here he has established equilibrium. With the trickiness he is able to covertly express his hostility and remain unharmed. When he is tricky, his eyes do not look open as they usually do; his chest is held and his shoulders are tighter. He is armored. However, in the presence of other children and with his family, he is still free and lively. He is able to wear his armor for special occasions only. This is temporary armoring.

Temporary armoring is a condition of survival in an armored society for all but the saintly. We are not always in a position to tell our boss that he is putting his work on our shoulders, or to tell our teacher that he has not prepared his lecture. We endure and bristle. So long as we can keep our bodies and spirits generally free, the temporary armoring does not cause serious harm. The danger is that temporary armoring may become chronic. Specific passive endurance may engender a generalized attitude of passive endurance, and we are in shackles.

Once the self-imposed restraint that protects us from an immediately threatening situation becomes converted to the security of the armoring, it takes an act of daring to break out and expand against our confines. If we lack that courage, we are caught and the imprisonment perpetuates itself.

There is a reciprocal relationship between what the psychoanalyst discovers and what the orgonomist observes. The unconscious material, the character attitudes and symptoms are the effects of the armoring process. Armoring is how the body and spirit becomes sick. The conventional psychiatrist deals with what the sickness consists of. To the extent that he recognizes only the initiating event in the environment and the symptoms which result, without awareness of the process by which the symptoms are formed, the psychiatrist is handicapped in reaching his patient.

Chapter 4
The Segmental Armoring

In arriving at a diagnosis the psychiatrist ordinarily observes this bit of aberrant behavior in the patient, adds it to subsequent diaplay of aberrant behavior and includes those parts of history that give evidence of emotional malfunction. We say cognitive function is disturbed to this extent, affect is inappropriate to this extent, ideation is altered to this extent; therefore, the patient is suffering from such and such.

Reich's procedure is different. Rather than list symptoms of illness, he first asks, "What is health?" To answer this complex question, we can begin with the fact that all living animals, including human beings, are comprised of cells which are made of protoplasm contained in a membrane. Flowing within the membrane, the protoplasm changes the shape of the cell in response to the environment. When the cell expands, protoplasm moves toward the environment, taking the membrane with it. When the cell contracts, protoplasm flows back toward the center of the cell, away from the environment. This flow of protoplasm toward and away from the environment is the natural pulsation of life. Pulsation results from the movement of energy through the cell -- energy Reich called "orgone." Its uninhibited movement, with the resulting plasmatic pulsation, is what Reich means by health.

Unhealthy, according to Reich, is just the opposite: a state of unhealth occurs when something interferes with the organism's free movement and natural pulsation. If we experiment with a single-cell organism, the amoeba, and expose it to noxious stimuli and hostile environments, we observe that as the environment begins to affect the amoeba, its membrane is no longer flexible. The protoplasm can no longer flow freely, and the pulsation of the cell is reduced. The cell is cut off from its natural, spontaneous functions.

Reich conceives of all animals, including man, as a protoplasmic bean-shaped mass confined in a membrane. He depicts the cephalic (head) end as larger to indicate more energy at that end.

In the case of a one-cell organism, we can directly observe the organism's pulsation. Multi-cellular organisms are composed of systems of separately pulsating components within the larger unitary pulsation. In the human organism, for example, there is the cardiac pulsation, the pulse of respiration (inspiration and expiration), the peristaltic pulse of the gastro-intestinal system, the pulse of the brain, the extensions and retractions of peripheral nerves. Moreover, each individual cell has its own pulsation. And all of this occurs within a large total organismic pulse. A deficiency of any of the smaller pulses from the cellular to the systemic level decreases the larger pulse. Thus, a constipated gastro-intestinal pulse puts a damper on the pulse of the total organism. The pulse of a heart with a defective valve affects the pulsation of the total organism. On the other hand, if the underlying pulse of the total organism is a shallow one, it must reflect on the systemic and cellular pulses within it. The quality of pulsation, then, is the basic criterion of health or disease.

Having established the significance of free pulsation (the free flow of energy) within the body, Reich discovered that there were seven segments where the energy could be blocked by armoring. With respect to armoring, the protoplasmic bean-bag can now be redefined as a shape with seven segments.

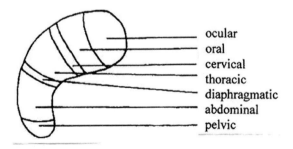

ocular
oral
cervical
thoracic
diaphragmatic
abdominal
pelvic

Reich defines these segments as "those organs and muscle groups which are in functional contact with each other, which can induce each other to participate in expressive movement." Each armor

37

segment is a functional rather that an anatomic unit. It corresponds to how emotions are expressed rather than where nerves, blood vessels, muscles, and organs lie anatomically. Blushing, for example, may be confined to the face and neck, not clearly delineated by anatomic structures.

A segment is the smallest unit capable of emotional expression. However, many segments may participate in a larger expression of emotion. For example, on one occasion a person may express anger by firing a withering look at the antagonist. On another instance, he may express a deeper anger with angry eyes and a roar through a snarled mouth, and may emphasize this anger with pounding fists and kicking feet.

With the exception of the arms and legs, which are appendages of the thoracic and pelvic segments, armoring always occurs at right angles to the longitudinal body axis. Armoring is a hardening and a tightening that limits the mobility of the affected parts and the free flow of energy along the head-to-toe axis.

The Ocular Segment

The eye segment comprises all the structures extending from the scalp to the base of the nose, upper cheeks and superior edge of the occiput (the occiput roughly comprises the very back of the skull). It contains some of the most important of the body's exteroceptors (the organs that sense the environment); the organs of vision, sound and smell; the cerebral hemispheres; the pituitary body with its important hormonal regulatory functions; the pineal gland; and the thalamus and reticular formation, which are key emotional regulators. It is because of the tremendous energetic exchange in this segment that we graphically represent the protoplasmic bean as expanded in the cephalic end. From the list of structures included within this segment, we can see that the functions served include intelligent action, awareness, concentration, extending outside oneself to experience the world by seeing, hearing, and smelling it, and, on the basis of these perceptions, regulating the organism's endocrine responses, autonomic functions, and body growth. Because the brain and its associated structures are included in this segment, and because there is more to be learned about brain functions, it is something of a black-box phenomenon. Unwittingly, when we work on this segment of armoring, we may produce some of the amazing physical changes that we observe in therapy.

For example, a patient in her thirties who had always had a straight torso (she had been nicknamed "slip-hips" by her high school friends when they discovered that she stuffed her skirts with slips to compensate for the lack of the natural feminine pelvic flare) noticed in the course of her therapy that her pelvic and hip contours were changing. Amazingly, at this relatively late time of life, she developed secondary sexual contours that she had always lacked. It was impossible to pinpoint exactly what therapeutic maneuvers were responsible for this change. But recent studies indicate that variations in environmental light intensity affect the time of pubescence of human females, an effect of a retinal-pineal pathway. It is conceivable that work on the patient's eye armoring had a pineal-stimulating effect which, in turn, resulted in this remarkable physiological change.

Except for the skin sensations and an as -- yet -- unexplored sense of the proximity of objects -- a sense which is most acutely developed in blind persons and the psychically gifted (but which is surely natural and not supernatural) -- the eye segment is the chief locus of all external perception. In emotional disorders, this segment is crucial in the patient relationship to other people and to the world. In the extreme examples, hysterical blindness and schizophrenia, the organs may totally fail to perceive. The patient with hysterical blindness, having faced a scene that is too traumatic to be borne by the psyche, becomes functionally blind. The schizophrenic in infancy sent his lively visual energy motherward and, failing to receive her warm visual response in return, learned -- by shutting off in his eyes -- to avoid the frustration of reaching out and feeling nothing. His eyes function sufficiently to prevent his bumping into objects, but all the lively, emotional uses of seeing are deadened. When he paints, his color is often intense and his forms exaggerated in an attempt to restore the life that has gone out of his eyes. When you look at his eyes and attempt to see him deeply, your eyes tend to become unfocused, as they do when looking at rippled water. When you try to make emotional contact -- your eyes to his -- you look and seek; he is not there. There is only space, and the configuration of an eye. It is interesting to note that a large proportion of the photographers and painters whom I have treated have had significant eye armoring. It would seem that these individuals had developed a skill involving seeing to compensate for the defective emotional uses of their eyes.

The schizophrenic makes minimal use of his eyes.[1] He sees only what is necessary for his physical safety and for going through the motions of living, so that he can withdraw his vision within his skull, where living is safer and more pleasant than in the real world.

My treatment room had been windowless; and after several years of working exclusively in artificial lighting, I had the exterior wall replaced with glass brick so that the room was lit by sun on clear days. A schizoid patient, who had come regularly since the pre-renovation period, walked into the treatment room one day, half a year after the glass bricks had been installed, and said, "Hey, what did you do to this room? It's different." I couldn't imagine how the room was changed since the previous week, and I answered that nothing was different. After an interval he said, "It's the wall; that used to be a solid wall." For six months he had worked in a room with natural, instead of electric light, and hadn't seen the difference.[2]

The schizophrenic is an extreme example, but most of us have lost some of the functioning potential of our eyes. As an exercise, patients are sometimes directed to look carefully at the individuals they pass in the street or at fellow passengers in the bus and to read the emotions on their faces. Typically the patient is eager for his next visit so that he can report his discovery. "They all look mad, or sad or bored, every one. I never saw that before. It's amazing."

Few of us look at one another; fewer still look openly and allow their eyes and faces to express what they feel. Mostly we use our eyes as a telescope to scan our environs. We stand behind the telescope. They can't see us.

The extent of the damage that is done to the individual through eye armoring is inestimable. The world experienced by brightly lit, lively eyes is a totally different place from the world viewed by those fortified behind their eyes. We are beginning to discover the price we pay in body functioning for armored eyes. A study[3] shows that

---

[1] A study by Leonard R. Proctor and Dominic W. Hughes in *Science*, Vol. 181, July 13, 1973, indicates that in a significant number of schizophrenic patients, smooth pursuit eye-tracking patterns "differ strikingly" from that of normals and non-schizophrenics. The probability of a perceptual dysfunction in schizophrenia is thus established outside of the treatment room.

[3] Lennon, Wm. and George H. Patterson: "Depth Perception of Sheep: Effects of Interrupting the Mother-Neonate Bond;" *Science*, Vol. 145, Aug. 21, 1964.

unmothered lambs have a significant deficit in depth perception compared with their mothered control peers. It is reasonable to expect that in time we shall discover the loss of other physical graces and synchronies, as well as the clumsiness of thinking, acting, and moving that is related to armoring in this segment.

Most of us have subconsciously noted the relationship between the eyes and intelligence. When we look at an individual for the first time, we note that he looks "bright" or "dull." His conversation may enhance or detract from the initial suggestion, but rarely is the basic impression incorrect. Anatomically the relationship between eye function and intelligence is clear since the optic nerve is a prolongation of actual brain substance. It is more than coincidence that when we understand, we say, "I see."

Problems of concentration, dissociation, depersonalization and consciousness are related to eye functions. All of the patients with idiopathic epilepsy (epilepsy of unknown origin, which includes the larger number of epileptics) whom I have examined have had severe problems of eye armoring. If we are aware, we can notice that as we drift toward sleep there is a physical movement upward and inward of the eyes into the skull. Any individual with problems of concentration has difficulty with the therapeutic exercises of following a darting object quickly. A tennis partner with heavy eye armoring constantly makes last minute dashes at the ball because his eyes do not go off until roused at the last moment by his brain.

An investigation of the varieties of optical perception makes semantic problems ("What did he mean by that?") seem simple in comparison. We never know what part of any situation others are "seeing." A schizophrenic patient reports that when he looks at his mirror image, the picture of himself evaporates and he sees only the outline of his body against the reflected walls. As we work persistently on her eyes, another patient comes to recognize that in emotional situations she picks out one detail in the scene and doggedly focuses on it to the exclusion of the gestalt. A third patient, when her eye functioning improves, recognizes that she had lived in a relatively monochromatic world until that time. A fourth patient always places his head askew when he looks at me. When I attempt to position my head parallel to his, he moves to maintain the skewed angle. From childhood he has had difficulties with numbers in series. He often mismeasures; and because he works in carpentry, his labor is unnecessarily burdened.

He lacks visual memory to the extent that if he closes his eyes he can barely remember what he has just seen.

None of these patients came to therapy because of visual problems. Each had symptoms which, so far as he or she knew, had no connection with armoring of the eye segment. Not invariably, but often, disorders of visual acuity, such as myopias, improve with work on this segment.

The eye is unique among the sensory organs in that it not only has receptive and coordinating functions, but is also an organ of expression. A devastating look can sometimes be more punitive that a physical blow. Eyes warm with understanding can do more to quiet pain than a chapter full of rationality. The energy discharged by vital eyes is powerfully effective and communicative. Just as so many eyes are crippled in their sensory functions, they are impaired expressively. The eyes should be able to fully state all emotions. The major emotions (rage, sadness, fear, joy, longing) as well as corollary expressions of affect (excitement, disdain, suspicion, questioning, flirtation, disappointment) all have their distinctive ocular expressions. The degree to which the eyes are incapable of expressing these emotions is an index of the extent of eye armoring.

Some individuals always wear a particular expression, hauteur for example, behind which they hide all other emotions, which they fear to express. Others walk about with blank eyes that communicate their own message: "I do not wish to be involved; please keep your distance." Social-worker eyes (a generalization, to be sure) say, "I care, I care," to cover, "Please, somebody love me," at a deeper level. Whenever a mask is worn as habitual demeanor, there is an accompanying set of eyes.

In the repression of some emotions, both the visual expression and the physiological concomitants of that expression are rendered non-functional. Thus, some patients begin to cry vocally and their eyes look sad, but there are no tears, or just a slight moistening in their eyes. "I haven't cried since I was child," they say. Not only has the desire to cry been banished, but the ability of the glands to produce tears has been destroyed. In the same way, when the eyes have less capacity to express lively emotion, the ocular muscles have less power to move the eye with alacrity.

The most common subjective symptom of armoring in the eye segment is headache. These headaches may be due to muscular tension in the frontal or, less frequently, in the parietal or temporal areas, or to suboccipital tension that radiates forward. An occasional headache does not indicate serious armoring in this segment, but recurrent headaches suggest the presence of chronic armoring. Various emotions may underlie the contraction in this area. The brows may be chronically knit in worry, or the forehead may be habitually raised as the eyes are widened in fear or tensed as the brow is contracted in pain.

In some anxious individuals the scalp is taut and tightly drawn; others, often with dead eyes, have scalps that sit slack on their skulls like loose skin.

Healthy eyes have a light that moves people and lifts spirits. Dull eyes have a draining quality.

The intimate relationship between the parts of an armored segment is illustrated by how the ears are sometimes deeply affected when the eyes go off. Several of my schizophrenic patients (whose eyes are badly armored) have recurrent complaints of ear disorder. One patient often pokes at an ear during the session, complaining that "something's wrong there." Another patient complained for weeks of severe ear pain. Examination by otoscope revealed no organic lesion. Auditory hallucinations are another indication of disordered ear function. They often occur concurrently with visual hallucinations. The clearest indicator of the eye-ear relationship occurs when the patient has been alert during the session and suddenly the eyes go out of contact completely. I address a remark to the patient at this time. When the eyes come back into contact, I question the patient on what I have just said. The patient looks surprised; he hasn't heard a thing. When the eyes went off, the ears did, too.

The disordered function of the sense of smell is more difficult to evaluate. Whether, in the process of evolution, the sense of smell has been so devalued, or whether the sense has suffered because of acculturation ("dirty" anal smells and "evil" genital odors), alterations of this sense do not appear with any great frequency in the examination of patients. To be sure, one sees patients with olfactory hallucinations, but more discrete, subtler alterations of function are only rarely observed.

Finally, some general comment about this segment: Long ago the eyes were described as "mirrors of the soul." The language may be antiquated but the observation is true. No segment of the body reveals so much character as the eyes. The sneaky, tricky, guilty, self-effacing, officious, mean, sad, bitter, cynical, scared, lively, ardent, hopeful, trusting, joyful qualities that combine to define the character structure can be read in the eyes. It is because eyes are so powerful that they are so widely avoided. To read eyes deeply is to be exposed to the pain, anger and dismay of our fellows, which is a heavy burden. On the other hand, deadened eyes can't look for long at bright eyes. They react as if the light were too bright. Sexuality is revealed in eyes as surely as in the pelvis -- not merely flirtatiousness or the momentary bright that the phallic character (the womanizer) flashes, but the revelation of how much energy one permits to flow in one's body, how deeply one lets oneself feel.

As a therapist, I notice armoring in the eye segment immediately. When I first greet the patient and elicit the chief complaint and the history, I observe the quality of the patient's eye contact. From that observation I arrive at a general evaluation of the relative dullness or liveliness of the patient's eyes. When the patient is on the couch, I test the ability of the eyes to express anger, sadness, fear, joy, suspicion or tenderness. The over-employment of any of these uses of the eyes -- for example, the constant side glancing of the eyes in a suspecting manner -- will help me to arrive at a diagnosis or begin to unravel the character structure. Various maneuvers test the patient's coordinative abilities. I may ask him to open his eyes wide, then to squeeze them shut, and to coordinate this with breathing. Individuals who have difficulty with concentration are unable to do this consistently over a long period. This test also may reveal that the patient has difficulty opening his eyes widely or shutting them tightly. While the patient lies on the couch, I may ask him to revolve his eyes around the walls as quickly as possible while still seeing. Careful observation reveals whether the patient is moving his eyes as a purely motor exercise, not visually sensing, or whether his eyes stick in a particular position, revealing distraction by a thought or simply turning-off. I may ask the patient to follow a finger darting within his visual field, or better, a flashlight. The inability of the eye muscles to perform reveals that the segment is armored.

The forehead and cheeks should be mobile. The patient should easily be able to make silly, frightened, angry, sad faces and to be serious in serious situations. Facial affect should be appropriate and proportioned.

The Oral Segment

The oral segment extends posteriorly from the chin to encompass the mouth, the jaw, the cheeks and the occipital muscles. It includes the upper reaches of the throat interiorly. Functionally these structures subserve all the uses of the vocal apparatus -- talking, crying, screaming, laughing. They include the functions of sucking, biting and grimacing. The character attitudes of the chin, jutting in pugnacity or slack in renunciation, are part of this segment.

Emotionally, the deepest expression of the oral segment centers on the ability to suck and the manner of sucking. Many of the other oral functions evolved in response to how the sucking needs were met in infancy. Constant, babbling loquaciousness, tight grinding jaws, a sullen facial expression, thin, taut lips, a tight voice -- these might never exist if the infant's oral needs had been completely gratified.

Although this segment is functionally unified, as illustrated by the fact that therapeutic work on the jaws often results in liberating energy in the mouth and lips, the oral segment well exemplifies the interrelatedness of armor segments. For example, some throat functions are within the anatomical limits of this segment and others within the next lower, cervical segment. Though a forward jutting chin is accomplished by the musculature of the oral segment, the retraction of the jaw is at least in part accomplished by the platysma of the cervical segment. Such facial expressions as anger cannot be completed without the participation of the ocular segment. For this reason, it may be impossible to elicit the repressed emotion in the oral segment until the armoring in the ocular segment has been worked through.

Besides pugnacity and slackness, the jaw participates in more subtle expressions. The slight raising of chin and lower lips expresses either doubt or disdain, depending on the accent. When the chin is lowered and the lower lip drawn downward and laterally, the expression is one of irony -- as if to say, the facts or events that have been witnessed do not fit any better than these parted, skewed lips.

There is a way of holding the jaw in a kind of squared configuration (I cannot describe it more graphically) that is habitual among some male homosexuals and less pronounced in some "butch" lesbians. It is so pathognomonic of the homosexual condition in some persons (though it is not a universal attribute of male homosexual facies) that one can diagnose homosexuality at a distance on the basis of this jaw configuration. For years I have tried unsuccessfully to fathom the meaning of the jaw-set. Anger and cynicism are in it, but there is a particular meaning in it which escapes me, and which I am sure is a key to homosexual character. A perceptive reader of the manuscript suggested that it represents a fierce fixation on the mother's nipple. This seems a valuable start.

Lips tell a tale both in their form and in the way in which they are held. There are the thick-lipped, agape-mouthed types that bespeak low-energy and mental defect. It is as if they lacked the will or energy to form their mouths. There are thin, tight, bitter lips; salacious lips which look crawly; lips which sit tightly against the teeth in a sneer ("No, thanks, I want no part of you or your food."); tense, beefy lips always waiting to be fed; and soft, rounded lips that can kiss sweetly and suck tenderly.

A frequent sight in our society is that of lips pursed in a vapid smile set against expressionless cheeks. The emptiness and lack of joy in this parody of a smile is obvious; yet it is prevalent. How can it be so transparent and, at the same time, so successful? -- for whatever exists and persists must, at some level, work. The answer is that most people have so much pain and sorrow and such deep fear of feeling and expressing it that by common consent we say, "I will pretend that you are happy if you pretend that I am happy." Smile, you're on Candid Camera.

The voice is an instrument for conveying messages. The message, though, does not lie in the verbalization alone but in the voice quality. The mumble-voice says, "I am talking to you from a greater distance and through a thicker wall than you know." The wobbly, thin voice says, "I am frightened." The frail voice, two registers too high says, "Though I look like a woman, I am a little girl." The voice that drones on in a monotone says, "Everything is dull; nothing excites me." The breathy voice says, "Do you remember the sounds of love-making?" The voice resolutely projected in barrel tones says, "I want you to think of me as a big, strong man."

The whine is a voice tone too commonly encountered. One hears it almost everywhere -- in patients, in social encounters, in actors. Whining could be the voice of our time. It expresses dissatisfaction and frustration, but mostly it expresses veiled anger. Whining is a way of annoying your mother while you give the appearance of suffering. Whiners are incapable of expressing their rage overtly, so they resort to this noisome vexation.

Tension in the throat makes most people speak at a higher frequency and with less modulation than is normal.

As a therapist, I ask the patient to sigh as she breathes. Her first attempts emerge as high and wispy sounds. She is instructed to visualize her throat as a big, wide, soft tube which carries deep sounds, and to lower her voice accordingly. The voice gets lower and lower as she sighs more freely and finally she hits a low resonant note full of feeling. Her mouth shapes into a smile of pleasure and she says, "There it is."

Each person has a "right" tonal range. The armored throats always vocalize outside that range. The unarmored voice varies constantly -- in pitch, volume, intensity -- so that it is a thing of interest and a pleasure to hear, even disregarding the words. A note on the interdependence of armor segments: although it is clear that the throat muscles and vocal cord tension are supremely important in the emotional expression of the voice, the breath power is supplied by the chest and diaphragm several segments lower.

The unarmored throat is sensitive to slight tactile pressures and the gag reflex is easily elicited. The infant is the model of the readiness to gag and vomit. When, after years of training, we learn to swallow our crying and screaming with our tense throats, we no longer gag as easily. We thrust a fistful of fingers into our mouths and touch and probe the back of our throat, but all that happens is that we salivate copiously. In other cases, each time that we begin to gag we hold our breath or cough. Armoring has blocked a simple, biological reflex.

Several years ago a patient with the proselytizing fervor of many new patients reported in his psychology class on his discovery in the course of his psychotherapy that he was unable to gag. The instructor and his classmates laughed with such hilarity that the class could not continue.

The jaws are frequently the locus of contained anger. At the time in an individual's history when the arms and legs are still too feeble to administer punishing blows, the power of the jaw musculature is sufficient to injure an offender. The threat of that power, as in a grimace which exposes the teeth, warns the antagonist of hostile intent. Repressed anger restrained in chronically taut jaw musculature is the agent of night-time tooth gnashing and other dental problems. When the tension is severe, the individual may develop a chronic low-grade pain in the jaws. Deep palpation in the angle of the jaw reveals the taut musculature and elicits the hypersensitive pain reaction. However, palpation is often not necessary to ascertain that the jaw is armored. Long practice makes the masseter muscles stand out in some individuals so that the diagnosis can be made on simple observation.

As a therapist, I can also determine the tension in the jaw by attempting to move the chin freely (opening and shutting the mouth) while the patient rests at ease. In some patients force is necessary to open, then to shut the mouth, despite the patient's best attempts to cooperate. After long armoring, only the patient can mobilize the jaw; it will no longer move easily, passively.

To evaluate mobility of lips and mouth, I request the patient to make faces. Where the segment is armored, the patient may have difficulty in moving the mouth in all positions or in moving the lips independently. The armored patient may be embarrassed by the lack of movement in his lips and may shamefacedly refuse the request to suck his thumb. Often the armored mouth reveals itself in a gradually accentuated perioral pallor as the patient breathes easily.

The varieties of sucking patterns reveal character as they illustrate specific armoring. Some suck so greedily that they would swallow their thumb if it were detachable. Others suck with the merest finger tip in their mouths. Some suck without involving their tongues, making little suction cups of their lips. Healthy, unarmored mouths make sensuous contact with the included finger and suck with efficient vacuum force but not avariciously.

The body has a special final place for holding crying that has passed the throat. This is the region of the submental triangle, behind the point of the chin. The tension of the muscles in this area, together with the tension in the deep neck muscles, is experienced as a "lump" in the throat.

The purple coloration of the face in the expression of rage indicates strong armoring in the neck segment; it is unnatural. The chronic plethoric coloration of the hypertensive and the alchoholic is also a mark of armoring.

In the unarmored face there should be no sharp lines of color or temperature demarcation. The skin (as in every segment) should have a vibrant quality. When the oral segment is free of armoring, it moves smoothly in making grimacing faces, silly faces, or angry faces, and participates with the eye segment in expressing wide-eyed, open-mouthed fear. It is capable of biting with force, but is not chronically contracted in a biting pattern. The voice reflects a throat free of tension, is capable of expressing fearful screaming, thundering rage, and sobbing that reaches to the belly; but it is always full, serious and modulated to express the nuances of all feelings. Sucking is easy and provides pleasure and peace. The skin responds to emotional states with appropriate color. The face flushes in the expression of anger and love, and grows pale when the body experiences fear.

The Cervical Segment

In the cervical segment, which covers the area of the neck, the superficial muscles are the platysma, trapezius and sternocleidomastoids, but the important armoring often centers in the deep neck musculature. The tongue is included in this segment because of its attachment to the hyoid bone, a part of the cervical osseous structure. The area also includes the throat, larynx, trachea, esophagus and thyroid gland.[4] The presence of the cervical and brachial plexi, the carotid arteries, jugular veins and vagus nerve, all in relatively exposed positions, creates the potential for serious disturbance with acute armoring and calls for therapeutic caution in approaching this segment. The function of armoring in the cervical segment is to hold back screaming and crying and to convert aggressive anger into stubborn resistance. The cervical segment is one of the chief body areas where the history of physical beatings in childhood is engraved.

I ask a young adult female patient to scream. "I can't," she answers timidly and with a trace of cuteness. "Do the best you can," I request. She tries, and emits a faint squeak. "Try again, and do it louder," I say. She tries, and with the same result. Pressing upon her tense cervical musculature, I urge her to try again. This time she utters a soft yell, followed immediately by a seizure of coughing and choking till the tears run from her eyes. She stretches her palms up as if to ward off a blow and her neck becomes doubly stiff.

The act of swallowing back the scream or the cry can easily be observed as the larynx bobs up and down. If the swallowing is forbidden, the patient reacts in one of three ways: He may quiet his

---

[4]Dew, R.: "The Biopathic Diathesis (Part VI: Hyperthyroidism)" *Journal of Orgonomy*, Vol. 7, No. 1, May, 1973.

respiration to the point where the impulse disappears, he may begin to cough or the gag or, if he is sufficiently courageous, he will scream or cry.

An arthritic woman in her forties, who barely speaks above a whisper and hasn't raised her voice in anger or crying for decades, lies on the couch in apparent distress. She looks brittle, as if the world is gradually impinging on her body space, imperceptibly, but slowly crushing her. Her appearance is so anguished that I, as a young therapist (this happened decades ago), am moved to do something to relieve the pressure. The holding in the throat is so strong and so obvious that I assumed that if I could free a little emotion from her throat she would be more comfortable. I apply pressure to the pipe-rigid neck, and she endures it stoically. I increase the pressure and urge her to react vocally. Finally a few tears drop from the corners of her eyes and she utters a soft cry. After a moment of this, she takes a rough, very deep breath and fails to exhale. Her eyes are staring and she is not breathing. Pressure on the chest and exhortations are to no avail. She continues to take these long, hoarse inspiratory breaths at what seems like minute intervals. She is beginning to become cyanotic. I call the police emergence squad to administer oxygen. The oxygen makes no difference; she still is not breathing. We decide to transport her to the nearest hospital for emergency consultation. Her color is still bluish but not deepening. The consultant can find no organic etiology for this state of affairs and comments that he never saw a patient with so little breathing, yet in no apparent danger. Her vital signs are within normal limits. We leave her in the care of a resident, who reports that over the span of a few hours her chest began to move more regularly, her color improved and quite matter-of-factly she asked if she could now go home.

Often, in eliciting a history, I ask "Do you ever cry?" The patient answers, "I cry all the time." When the patient is on the couch and cries, it is an exaggerated whine through an armored throat. It bears little resemblance to full, deep crying. It represents the spill over of the repressed grief that never gets released, just as constant irritability and bitchiness represent the overflow of unreleased rage.

Deep crying, though it is ultimately liberated through the throat, has its origin in the diaphragmatic region and surfaces downward to the abdomen and upward through the wide open throat and mouth. When one cries or screams fully, one is the vessel of the emotion. The crying comes in waves that may increase in intensity at the beginning, then gradually decrease with time. To the extent that one observes oneself crying or alters the sound or intensity, the crying is not free. Despite the intensity of the pain, which is at the source of the crying, the full surrender to the impulse is satisfying. There is exhilaration in the freedom to give in to one's energetic flow.

Because of the habit of clamping the throat against the sound of intense emotions, it is frequently physically painful for patients to attempt to scream. The throat automatically constricts against the emerging sound; and after a few attempts, the patient cannot go on because of the pain. When the throat is unarmored, then one may scream for long periods without discomfort. The only physical consequence may be a temporary slight deepening of the voice.

Chronic constriction in the neck is related to the tendency to faint (because of pressure on the carotids) and to the fear of fainting and of being throttled (the physical sensation of constriction is converted in suitable subjects to the fantasied choking). The fear of choking, in turn, is related to some fears of being crowded ("I will not be able to catch my breath."). The hypertensive with the reddish face is holding in his neck so that the circulation from his head is blocked-off. The terrible-tempered, purple-faced despot has attained his coloration by virtue of acute cervical armoring, which tightens to contain his deepest rage. Because of this armoring, he often "chokes with rage." The cervical armoring, together with oral blocking, has been implicated by Dew in the etiology of hyperthyroidism.[5]

The compulsive individual may manifest cervical armoring which is centered not so much in the deep throat muscles as in the muscles which control turning or tilting the head. He holds his head rigidly straight; and when you attempt to turn his head to right or left, there is great resistance. This armoring has evolved in part from his need to travel the straight and narrow path. He cannot permit himself the dangerous possibility of straying, and his neck-set performs the same function as blinders on a horse.

The same armoring is present in those who are hypersensitive to sudden turns and twists, reacting with dizziness and nausea (assuming, of course, that there is no disorder of the cerebellum or inner ear).

---

[5] *Ibid.*

The rigid compulsive patient is sitting on the edge of the couch. I ask him to move his neck, shoulders and arms as freely as he can. With his best efforts he can move his head only to a position about 30° from forward, and he moves as if his head were mounted on a ratchet. I work on the posterior cervical musculature, then move the patient's head side-to-side at a larger angle. I then request the patient to try again. Now his head revolves wider and easier, but he soon stops. He says, "I can't do that, it makes me sick to my stomach."

The main cause of armoring of the posterior cervical musculature, however, is stubbornness. The armoring conveys two messages. On the deepest level it represents the inability to give in to the rage that is present, and on the more superficial level it says, "You cannot hurt me or push me further; I will not yield." For some persons who are unable to actively oppose, it is the only available means of opposition. If the reader will play at being stubborn, he will note how these neck muscles automatically stiffen. Cervical armoring is the signature of stubbornness.

There is another possible meaning in this armoring. Individuals who have been physically beaten in their childhood, or those to whom the environment administered a symbolic beating, learn to harden themselves against the blow and against their reactive rage by tightening their necks and attempting to reduce its surface area. In some this becomes a chronic attitude of withdrawal and their necks grow that way permanently.

And finally there is the cervical armoring of the haughty -- those who attempt to make themselves high. Here the neck musculature appears as if stretched, the superficial muscles, especially in older persons, standing out beneath the skin as taut strands of ropes. The attempt here is to create as much distance as possible between the spiritual head and the benighted body, especially its naughty nether parts. Such necks must never surrender softly, lest the body sensations pervert the lofty brain.

The unarmored cervical segment is capable of crying, screaming and raging freely; vocal sounds are resonant and emotionally responsive. The esophagus is free to participate in the gag reflex. The neck is capable of free, coordinated and graceful movement and participates with shoulder movements in a harmonious manner. Palpation reveals no inordinate muscular tension.

The Thoracic Segment

The thoracic segment extends from below the neck to the diaphragm. The musculature involved includes the pectoralis major and minor, the deltoids, the serratus, the intercostals, the trapezius, latissimus dorsi, the rhomboids, infra-spinatus and other smaller muscles and the deep fascia. If any segment were to be considered more important than another (though if we are examining complete emotional and physical functioning such a consideration is merely an intellectual exercise), it would be the thoracic segment, for two reasons: First, because it contains organs absolutely vital to the life process -- the heart and lungs. Second, because it is the chief motor source of the body's energy level. Thus, armoring in this segment affects the function of every others segment. In addition to the heart and lungs, this segment contains the esophagus, which is significant because it is apparently the locus (possibly with the lower end of the trachea) of the "knot" in the chest, and also because it participates in the gag reflex.

All patients who come to therapy exhibit some degree of armoring of the chest segment. In some, the chest may be granitic from years of constraint; in other, the only difficulty may be in the amplitude or completeness of the respiratory excursions. The fact that every patient has an armored chest does not imply, however, that an unarmored chest is tantamount to health. Theoretically it is possible for the chest to be unarmored and for armoring to be present in other segments, particularly lower ones. But in the course of everyday life it would be unlikely because of the dynamics of chest armoring, i.e., if there is armoring in another segment, it is likely that the chest, too, would be armored to decrease the energetic push against the armored segment.

To live one's life with a totally free chest implies the ability to feel fully, to immerse oneself in the currents of existence with daring and energy, and generally, to be free of armoring. For wherever there is armoring elsewhere in the body, the chest segment comes to the aid of that armoring by reducing the intensity of the energetic input, thus ameliorating the pain. if one represses a scream, the armored chest has assisted in that process by braking the general energy level, making it less likely that one would feel like screaming. If the healthy newborn is subjected to long separations from its mother, as it is in a typical American hospital, there is "increasing and persistent muscular tension and this increasing tension is accompanied by inadequate breathing," as Margaret Ribble[6] noted in her study of 600 newborns. If the vicissitudes of life induce some to turn away by not seeing, chest armoring comes to the aid of the eye armoring by dampening the life fires, making their lives a walk-through part.

By reducing the energy level, chest armoring makes all pain less acute, all conflict less tense. Unbearable situations tend to become more tolerable. Chest armoring begins in early infancy when the neonate discovers the tension-alleviating properties of deep inspiration followed by incomplete expiration. Later, at the age at which objects of fear can be recognized, the child reacts with the deep drawn intake of breath, which becomes part of the pathognomonic reaction to fear. In a society in which the needs of infants and children are so poorly met, in which conformity is so valued, the prevalence of chest armoring is no surprise.

One of the more acute manifestations of chest armoring occurs in the anxiety syndrome. Here not only does the therapist see the chest held in fear of exposing the repressed emotion, but the patient also perceives the armoring and lists it among his symptoms. "I can't catch my breath." "I get this knot in my chest." "My chest feels as if there's a weight on it."

The hypertensive patient always has an armored chest. Whether the chest held in chronic expansion is etiologic in the hypertensive disorder or whether the same pathology constricts the blood vessels as it constricts the chest is difficult to say. The relationship of chest armoring to heart disease is highly suggestive, but at this point is incompletely elucidated. Dew[7] has made valuable contributions to the consideration of chest armoring and its relationship to arteriosclerosis and coronary artery disease.

Disorders of the respiratory apparatus -- emphysema, bronchial asthma, chronic bronchitis, chronic obstructive pulmonary disease, bronchogenic carcinoma -- are associated with specific configurations of chest armoring. Dew[8] has described these connections and once again the interested reader is referred to the original articles for detailed articulation of these processes.

---

[6]Ribble, M.: *Infantile Experience in Relation to Personality Development in Personality and Behavior Disorders*, J. McV. Hunt, Ed. R. Hunt, Co. NY, 1944.
[7]Dew, R.: "The Biopathic Diathesis (Part IV, Arteriosclerosis and Coronary Artery Disease)," *Journal of Orgonomy,* Vol. 4, No. 2, Nov. 1970.
[8]Dew, R.: "The Biopathic Diathesis (Part V, The Pulmonary Biopathies)," *Journal of Orgonomy,* Vol. 6, Nos. 1 and 2, May and Nov., 1972.

Aside from its function as energy inhibition, the armoring of the chest also clamps down on the strongest expressions of love, rage, sadness and longing, as well as fear. It is not by chance that the popular imagination links the heart and emotions of love. The lover in the throes of his passion recognizes that sensation in his chest which we call love. In fact, his ignorance of anatomy and perhaps his preoccupation with his love object betray him. What he perceives as the pleasant affection of his "heart-shaped" heart is actually the suffusion of pleasurable sensation from the coeliac plexus (solar plexus), which lies beneath his diaphragm. The sensation spreads upwards from the plexus through the chest and downward through the abdomen toward the genitals. And, in the course of experiencing these delicious sensations, the lover's chest heaves with rapture, as the old writers used to say.

The complete expression of any deep emotion is accompanied by the same wide excursions of the chest. The chest surges with longing. It pants with rage and it convulses in billows with sobbing. Conversely, it is held as rigidly as possible when these emotions must be repressed. As hot rage is characterized by the heaving chest, cold rage is described by the held chest, the taut tense exterior with the fire burning deep within.

The central role of chest armoring -- as an energy inhibitor and as a clamp on deep emotions -- is the reason that breathing figures so predominantly in psychiatric orgone therapy. Free and open breathing energizes the body and accentuates the areas of armoring, calling them into play by increasing the energetic pressure. New patients are often amazed at the inner turmoil a few full breaths can bring up.

I ask the patient who is on the couch for the first time to breathe according to my instructions. She is a shy, severely inhibited young lady with pronounced symptomatology. Seeking relief from the pain, she follows the instructions diligently. After a dozen breaths, tremors appear, first in her jaw, then in her shoulders, and soon she is all atremble. She feels strong currents going through her torso and extremities. "What are you doing to me?" she asks. "Is this bed hooked up to anything?" and she looks around for wires. "No wires, no connections," I say, "that's all from your breathing." "You mean just taking those few breaths did this? Would the same thing happen if I did it at home?" "It would if you did it the same way, but you had better not try it yet without supervision," I advise.

There is often interest in the relationship between unarmored breathing and the breathing prescribed in yoga exercises. They are quite different, both in the mechanics and in effect. Yoga breathing entails inspiring deeply and exhaling a long, controlled breath, and its object is control. The breathing in therapy entails moderately deep inspiration with uncontrolled expiration; the emphasis is on the complete and uninhibited release of the inspired air. Its object is-- the exposure to freedom and the abandonment of control mechanisms -- the opposite of the yogic object.

The breathing mechanism may be disturbed in either its inspiratory or expiratory phases. In individuals who breathe very shallowly, the inhibition to expire may not be apparent until in the inspiratory phase is increased. The reason is that with minimal breathing there is no cause for inhibition. So little oxygen has been taken in, the fires burn so low, that nothing is stirred-up; there is just enough energy to maintain existence. When the patient is asked to breathe more deeply, a marked distortion appears in the expiratory phase.

I request a new patient who is breathing superficially to breathe more deeply. After a few breaths, he begins to clear his throat on almost every expiration. I admonish him to stop this, and he does. He then pushes each breath out, as if exhaling operated on the piston principle. I instruct him to fill his chest and to let it collapse without any impetus. He proceeds to inspire deeply, raising and tightening his shoulders and constricting his neck at the top of each inspiration. I work on the exposed cervical armoring, digging my fingers into the tight musculature.

I request another barely-breather to breathe more deeply, and he increases his breathing in scarcely perceptible increment. I encourage wider breathing by applying pressure to the sternum with each expiration and supplementing this with work on the intercostals in the region of the axilla. Now the patient is breathing more deeply, and for a few moments his breathing is less inhibited. "This feels good, Doc," he says. He looks more alive and is clearly enjoying this new status; but he cannot maintain it for long, for now his diaphragmatic armoring comes into play and his belly begins to balloon with each expiration.

From a therapeutic point of view, uninhibited breathing may be examined in two ways. The narrower aspect concerns its energizing function. The broader view incorporates the awareness that with totally free expiration comes an energetic impulse that, if unimpeded, flows through the abdomen and is perceived in the genitals. This aspect of respiration has no direct connection to the air-breathing function of respiration. It is the reason that individuals armor against free breathing in segments below the chest. As chest armoring decreases in therapy, the armoring in lower segments increases to ward off the sensations of the anxiety-provoking energy as it courses to the genitals.

A quotation from a patient who was beginning to learn to breathe fully on expiration is indirectly pertinent to this phenomenon. She said, "Breathing all the way down makes you feel as if you have legs. When I was a child I never felt my legs; they weren't as if they were anesthetized, but as if they were just hanging there."

Another patient said, "When I breathe all the way down and it's soft down there I get the feeling that I'll be swept away, and I have to hold on."

Others are not able to define the difficulty so exactly. One patient working on breathing says, "I don't want to do this. I don't want to feel this," and she proceeds to cry.

Diminishing discomfort by inhibiting respiration is a process that starts in infancy. The child holding its breath is attempting to establish a modus vivendi; some body sense is aware that in the face of unbearable pain, holding the breath as long as possible will block the pain. For lesser pain, the prescription is not as dramatic; one need merely impede the completion of expiration.

Patients exhibit many varieties of the inhibition to breathe out completely. There is the expiration in two parts, in jerks, the half or three-quarter expiration, the propulsive expiration, and the expiration with sudden brakes.

We have been speaking of the relationship of respiration to the regulation of one's own emotions. Respiration also relates the individual to his world. In deep inspiration we take in the world, in an almost literal sense. And in full expiration we abandon ourselves to a cosmic stream. Insofar as we are afraid of life or fearful of other people, we cannot risk free breathing.

In addition to the respiratory function, the thoracic segment includes the muscular activity of the shoulder girdle and upper extremities. The chief armoring function of the shoulder girdle is to activate the defensive armor plate of the scapula, clavicle and shoulder musculature. With fear or anxiety, a person tends to compress the dorsal musculature and raise the shoulders, as if to ward off blows from behind and protect the neck.

I instruct a patient who has problems expressing aggression to yell at me offensively, making an angry face. At first her attempts are totally ineffectual, but with encouragement and direction the emotion of anger begins to come through. With the expression of hostility, her shoulders rise until her skull is turtled into the shell of her shoulders.

The armoring of the musculature of the upper extremities involves either the inhibition of aggression or of reaching out with tenderness and longing.

I direct a well-built, muscular man in his forties to hit the couch angrily, with all his might. I observe that each time he punches, he reduces the velocity in his swing just before contact, so that the blow is merely a soft tap. The patient recognizes the validity of these observation and determines to try harder. The second attempt results in the same soft taps. Try as he may, he cannot punch hard.

I direct a young man to reach out with his arms, breathe fully and easily and call, "Mama" as he reaches. "Christ, Doc, that's silly," he says. "Let's do something else." I insist, and he makes an embarrassed attempt, breaking into smiles, then laughter. His hands turn in on themselves, and I direct him to stretch the fingers out and reach as he continues. His voice becomes more convincing, but his hands keep turning inward or his arms bend at the elbows. I persist in requesting complete reaching out; and when, after a while, he finally does it, the expression on the young man's face becomes serious and intense. he starts to cry, then sob.

At first one may be reminded of group sensitivity sessions in which participants are encouraged to punch pillows to release repressed hostility. They punch and punch, and except for the value of the activity as exercise, they achieve nothing because each of them punches in his usual inhibited manner. The key to the therapeutic uses of aggressive activities lies in discovering the emotional roots in the inhibition.

I engage in playful boxing with a young adult female patient. Despite my assurance that I will not hurt her, she cannot bring herself to move her arms from their protective position in front of her face. In spite of my verbal prodding, she cannot make the slightest aggressive movement. I continue to poke at her defensive position and, helpless, she begins to cry. This activity is a symbolic recreation of her lifelong reaction to others' aggression.

The inhibited aggression in the armored upper extremities is revealed not only in the larger shoulder and arm movement but in tense finger movements, such as constantly drumming and twittering fingers or restless hands.

I walk to the waiting room to call in the next patient. She is an early middle-aged woman with severe arthritis of the shoulders and neck. Superficially she is always pleasant and passively cooperative. She is knitting and so absorbed in the process that she is unaware of my presence. I watch her fingers as they work, and I gain a new appreciation of Madame Lafarge knitting by the guillotine.

Just as the expression of hate and rage is inhibited in the hands and fingers, so is the manifestation of tenderness. There are persons whose touch is as gross as rough bark. They are unable either to perceive tenderly through their finger tips or to transmit tenderness. This also is armoring.

With pronounced blocking of energy in the extremities, as in the thoracic armoring that accompanies anxiety, the hands are cold and moist with cold sweat. This effect is so pronounced that it has become a sign for detecting anxiety.

Armoring of the paraspinal musculature (muscles along the spine) in the thoracic as well as in lower segments has the function of converting rage into spite. If the reader will pretend to feel spiteful, he will notice how these muscles along the spine tighten automatically. In a less intense mode, armoring of these same muscles accompanies interpersonal withdrawal.

Armoring of the thoracic segment is evident in the skin tone, color changes, temperature changes, skin sensitivity and tissue sensitivity within this area. The sensitivity of female breasts is, of course, more significant than the sensitivity of the male pectoral area.

Armoring of respiration can be visually observed. Abnormal tension in the paraspinal and shoulder area is established by palpation and observation of abnormal carriage. Armoring affecting the aggressive uses of the upper extremities is elicited when the patient attempts to punch, pinch, throttle or scratch. Ticklishness to any marked degree and an irritability to touch in the thoracic region are indices of armoring in this area.

The free chest looks soft and alive. It is free of any tension at the bottom of expiration, and the shoulders move forward gently in an expression of yielding as the neck and head flex backward softly and subtly.

The Diaphragmatic Segment

The diaphragmatic segment occupies the body region between the thoracic cavity superiorly and the abdominal cavity inferiorly. The diaphragm arises from the xiphoid process (the lower-most portion of the breast bone) of the sternum anteriorly, the lower six ribs on either side and, posteriorly to the first and second lumbar vertebrae on the left and the first, second and third lumbar vertebrae on the right. It lies in close association to the pericardium, esophagus, stomach, duodenum, liver, gall bladder, kidneys, pancreas and spleen. From the point of view of therapy, probably its most significant anatomic relationship is to the coeliac plexus (solar plexus).

On a purely physiological-anatomic level, the diaphragm is used in all expulsive efforts, whether sneezing, crying, coughing, laughing, vomiting, excreting feces or urine or expelling the fetus from the uterus. From the naming of these expulsive acts, it is apparent that the energies of the diaphragm may be expended either upward to the cephalic end or downward to the caudal end. In infants one can sometimes observe the simultaneous discharges of the diaphragm in either direction as the infant vomits and defecates at one swoop. In therapy one occasionally observes the same free play of the diaphragm when the patient vomits propulsively and passes flatus.

The close relationship of the diaphragm to the heart and to a host of abdominal viscera would indicate that armoring in this segment may be accompanied by a number of organic disorders. Clinical practice confirms this.[9] The diaphragm pointed toward the head is

---

[9]Nelson, A., "The Diaphragmatic Block," *Journal of Orgonomy*, Vol. 6, Nov. 1972.

associated with vomiting; and vomiting is a physiological expression of disgust ("I cannot stomach this"). The diaphragm poised for discharge at the caudal end, as in diarrhea, is obviously related to rage at an anal level. It is therefore not surprising that armoring of the diaphragm may contain explosive rage going back to infantile levels.

The chief significance of the diaphragmatic segment in therapy (and here is its uniqueness) is not what emotions are contained when the segment armors, but what happens when, with the segments above it , it is free of armoring. At this point we leave the realm of words that we use to describe emotions and enter the province of biological functioning. No word conveys the phenomenon that occurs when the patient, unarmored from head through diaphragm, breathes through the entire body freely. What happens is a series of waves of pleasurable sensation that move toward the pelvis, accompanied by a folding of the upper abdomen so that the upper torso and pelvis approximate one another while the head and neck fall back in a yielding posture. The closest word that describes this occurrence is surrender. But we must remember that the word is several dimensions removed from the phenomenon per se.

Armoring in the diaphragmatic segment is revealed in catching at the bottom of the expiratory breath and in ballooning of the abdomen with expiration. There is frequently a spinal lordosis (arching of the lower back) present; the space between the patient's back and the surface of the couch easily contains the breadth and width of the therapist's hand. The muscular tension responsible for the lordosis is revealed in the patient's hypersensitivity to deep palpation and in the ropiness of the muscles of the back.

The maneuver most closely associated with diaphragmatic armoring is gagging. The receptors in the throat form the afferent end of the reflex, and the diaphragmatic impulse the efferent end. Whereas at the oral end the gagging may be distorted by a variable play of the throat muscles or conversion of gagging to coughing, at the diaphragmatic level the only variability is in the intensity of the diaphragmatic contraction. In eliciting the gag reflex the most

---

1   Dew, R.:" The Biopathic Diathesis (Part VIII, Gastrointestinal Peptic Ulcer)," *Journal of Orgonomy*, Vol. 7, No. 2, Nov. 1973.
2   Levy, N.: " Hepatitis as a Complication of Therapy," *Journal of Orgonomy*, Vol. 4, May 1970.

important provision is that the patient breathe freely and continuously while gagging.

When such a basic reflex as the gag reflex is lost, there must be a significant cause. The fact that the reflex is impaired in so many individuals makes the case even more intriguing. In what cause have we sacrificed a biological reflex?

Reich[10] found the clue in the course of treating a patient. He observed that when a patient repeatedly exhaled fully, he developed such hypersensitivity of the lower abdomen and pelvic region that he reacted by holding his breath. Each time Reich touched the sensitive area, the patient reacted with a start. But when the patient continued to breathe down through the whole body, his sensitivity to touch disappeared; when he held his breath again, the sensitivity returned. This phenomenon could be repeated at will.

The hypersensitivity in the patient's abdominal and pelvic segments is clearly related to an inability to tolerate sexual sensation; this obtained only when he held his breath and tensed his diaphragm. When the diaphragm was coaxed to the unarmored condition and the patient breathed into his pelvis, he could tolerate the sexual sensations. Conversely, with the diaphragm armored, he stopped the sexual flow but he felt tension and reflex irritability (an analogue of anxiety). In the act of balancing between anxiety and sexuality, the diaphragm played a critical role.

A question poses itself at this point: How does the diaphragm balance anxiety and sexuality? An examination of the functional anatomy of the area provides a plausible answer. First, the diaphragm is a powerful muscle. We have already seen how, when the diaphragm functions without tension, it is characterized by propulsive responses (sneezing, vomiting, diarrhea). On the other hand, when it is tense it constitutes a pretty powerful bundle of tension. Second, it is near the solar plexus, the largest of the sympathetic nerve plexi. Because of the proliferation of organs beneath the diaphragm, tremendous energy flows in this area. Given a system which discharges a large quantum of energy (the solar plexus) and a system capable of blocking off a great deal of energy (the diaphragm), the ability of the diaphragmatic segment to release or inhibit energy flow to lower segments is comprehensible.

To reiterate: The armored diaphragm may serve to bind deep rage; it may also limit crying to a tolerable level. When it functions in

---

[10]Reich, W., *The Function of the Orgasm*, The Noonday Press, N.Y., 1961, page 3.

this manner, the crying is characterized by repeated short jerks within one expiration, rather than the inspiratory-expiratory heaving of the full cry. But its largest function in armoring is to bind energy that would be intolerable to the subject if perceived and experienced. The fact that people spontaneously point to this area when speaking of overwhelming emotions confirms this use of the armored diaphragm.

Armoring in the diaphragmatic segment is revealed by an inability to breathe to the full completion of expiration, by ballooning of the abdomen with expiration, by the inability to vomit with gagging, by lordosis of the spine, excessive ticklishness of the diaphragmatic region, spasmodic crying, holding in this region when expressing anger and by the inability to perceive pleasurable sensation in the subdiaphragmatic areas of the body with full, free breathing.

The Abdominal Segment

The abdominal segment extends from below the diaphragm to the brim of the pelvis. The musculature includes the external oblique muscles and their aponeuroses, the internal oblique muscles, the transversus abdominis and rectus abdominis, all of these located anteriorly and laterally; the sacrospinalis, quadratus lumborum and psoas major and minor muscles, located posteriorly. The abdominal segment contains the larger portion of the intestines, the lower edges of the kidneys, the ureters, and the portions of the uterus and urinary bladder.

People hold their abdomens tight mostly from fear. When the abdominal armoring is attacked, fear is the first emotion, then the rage that is always covered by fear. The two areas where fear of physical assault reside are the back of the neck (from apprehension of a possible blow to the head)) and the abdomen (from apprehension to the belly). A.S. Neil,[11] the founder of the Summerhill School, was fond of classifying his charges into the "stiff bellies" and the "soft bellies," roughly the fearful and the self-assured.

To a lesser extent, the fear of physical attack also resides posteriorly, in the lumbar musculature. The common expression of armored loin muscles is the tension of spite. However, in my experience, the spite contained in the shoulder and neck armoring exceeds that of the abdominal segment. Often tension occurs in the flank region in those who are relatively unarmored but have not had the

---

[11]Neil, A.S., *The Free Child*, Herbert Jenkins, LTD, London, S.W., 1953

opportunity for genital discharge over a long time. This tension usually disappears when the sexual needs are gratified.

The therapist recognizes abdominal armoring when there are temperature or color demarcations over the surface of the area, when there is superficial or deep muscular tension in the area, when the abdomen blocks the wave of excitation that originates in the diaphragmatic segment when the patient breathes down into the pelvis, when there is excessive ticklishness of the flank musculature or when somatic[12] illness in the segment reflects the armoring.

We had been working on breathing-through the whole body without resistance and the patient was getting the knack. She first felt generally pleasurable sensations flowing in her abdomen, then more specifically genital sensations, which she enjoyed at first but soon terminated by holding her chest. She reported that she couldn't go on because the picture of her father suddenly appeared in her head, and thereafter the sensations became scary.

When she arrived for her next visit, she looked as if she were privy to some great secret. "Boy, do I have something to show you," she said, as she passed me at my desk and moved into the treatment room.

As I observed her on the treatment couch, there was a rosy rash starting in a line across the middle of her abdomen. "See that?" she said, "It's a red light; it says 'Stop!'"

The Pelvic Segment

The pelvic segment consists of all the structures below the pelvic brim, including the lower extremities. Most of the pelvic musculature is involved in the armoring of this segment, but among the most frequently involved muscles are the levator ani, the anal sphincters, the bulbocavernosus, the ischiocavernosus (which regulate erection of the penis and clitoris), the gluteal muscles and the thigh adductors.

The pelvic segment contains the uterus and ovaries, the male reproductive apparatus, the external genitalia, the urinary bladder, the urethra and the distal portion of the intestinal tract with the rectum and anus.

---

[12]Dew, R., "The Biopathic Diathesis (Part VII: Gastrointestinal Peptic Ulcer)," *Journal of Orgonomy*, Vol. 7, No. 2, Nov., 1973.

In this culture, armoring of the pelvic segment is practically universal. If the pelvis had escaped armoring with the prohibitions of toilet training in the anal stage, it could hardly avoid the pleasure-dampening effect of a love-negative culture several years later. In this context it is appropriate to mention that the apparent relative sexual freedom of contemporary adolescents must not be confused with sexual health. While it is obvious that there is more sexual activity in adolescence than heretofore, and while this is generally to be preferred over abstinence, the greater part of adolescent sex is of the "balling" and "screwing" variety, a long distance from healthy loving. So we do not anticipate that the generation of the children of our children will be free of pelvic armoring.

The armored pelvis lacks life. When it engages in the genital embrace, it does so in a way that is business-like, or perfunctory, or athletic, or pretending-to-feel-what-it-doesn't, or hateful, or pornographic, or little, or scratch-an-itch, or that says I expect-this-to-be-a-soul searing, earth-shaking experience. The sex-researchers (and I am not demeaning the value of their research, but describing the point from which they start) and the sex professors, like most of the rest of us, have armored pelves.

The main function of the armored pelvis is to avoid the full sensation of the flow of energy into the genitals. In attaining this end, the anus is chronically constricted, or if the tension is not chronic, it constricts acutely and is pulled back by the levator muscles as sexual excitement increases. The pelvis tends to be held in a retracted position. The buttocks are tensed and often cold. The thigh adductors are tense, tending to hold the legs together. The pelvic floor is drawn up. The penis inclines to a cyanotic bluish coloration in some cases; and though one does not inspect the vaginal mucosa in therapy, there is a high probability of a similar tendency in some females.

One occasionally sees another kind of dead pelvis characterized by an appearance of utter flaccidity and flabbiness.

When the individual with an armored pelvis is requested to move his pelvis, he tends to move legs, pelvis and abdomen in one piece, as if they were plastered together. The side-to-side pelvic movement (the pelvic "no") is much easier for him to achieve than the independent back and forth pelvic tilt (the pelvic "yes").

The downward wave-like sensations achieved by freeing the upper segments of armoring are stopped as by a wall at the pelvis.

There is either total anesthesia for the pleasurable sensations, or they are perceived minimally, and as their intensity increases, so does anxiety.

A patient who has endured pelvic anxiety for months in therapy, but who has been free of her acute anxiety attacks for more than a month, reports that the degree of sexual pleasure with her husband exceeds anything she had known. In the midst of this halcyon period, she calls from work for an emergency appointment. When she arrives she is pale, but not as badly shaken as in the past. "It happened again," she says, "and I thought that maybe I was through for good. It started down here (pointing to pelvis) and it gradually rose to my head and I started to get nutty, and then it started to go downward and when it got to there (pelvis), I got so scared I thought I would faint. So I sat down on a step and called my assistant."

Another young lady working through pelvic armoring says, "I was having sex and it was better than it's ever been, and suddenly something happened that I think felt good, but I got so scared that I opened my mouth to scream, and I was so dammed scared that nothing came out."

Anxiety is the hallmark of pelvic armoring. The anxiety comes from acute fear of strong pleasure. Behind this anxiety is a rage from being denied what could feel so good. Rage and contempt sometimes speak directly in the hardness with which some people "make love"; the general, unconscious, cultural awareness of this hardness is revealed in the ever-present, "Fuck you."

Chapter 5
The Physical Dissolution of Armoring

A chapter on reducing armoring should be introduced with a warning that the techniques described are intended neither as a do-it-yourself, self-improvement program, nor as procedures with which psychotherapists untrained in orgonomy should experiment. Many of the techniques demand that the therapist be open and unarmored in the particular segment upon which he is working. An armored therapist using a particular technique in cookbook fashion would, in most cases, be ineffective. Or he might even increase the armoring that he is seeking to remove. The worst possibility is that he might create problems that he is not prepared to deal with.

These techniques are not things in themselves; they are used by the orgonomist at a certain time, according to a particular intuition and often with a deviation from the way they are described in writing. If the practice of medicine is an art as well as a science, the practice of orgonomy is that art carried to an exponential power. There is no finite body of therapeutic maneuvers. The therapist is always improvising, creating, working in accordance with his own structure and energy at that time. The critics and writers who have described the physical maneuvers of orgonomy as manipulation or massage are completely off the mark.

The Ocular Segment

The physical approach to the ocular segment is determined by what is being repressed, where in the segment the block is located and how it is being held. For example, in a patient with constant apprehension and frequent headaches, we may note that the eyebrows and forehead are chronically raised in a low-level expression of fear and worry. We might then apprise the patient of what we see and ask him to consciously exaggerate this expression so that he may feel what he is doing. Work on wide-eyed fear over many sessions might eventually put him in touch with an acute fear that had been repressed and forgotten. Or direct work on the eye fear may be too threatening for him to deal with at that time and he may resist with angry determination, revealed in increasing spasticity of his jaws. We might then temporarily shift our focus to the angry jaw and confront the anger before resuming the work on the fear in the eyes.

The therapist finds tension in the scalp directly by palpation. More subtle tension, usually located in the temporal, parietal and suboccipital areas, is revealed when the patient is hypersensitive to pressure. To elicit the emotion that is bound by this tension, the therapist painfully kneads these areas until the patient expresses anger, fear or crying.

"Hey, don't do that. What are you trying to do, break my head? I know there's something wrong in there; otherwise I wouldn't be here (giggle). How long do you intend to keep that up? . . . You having fun? Go ahead if that's how you get your kicks . . . . Man, are you some kind of sadist? . . . That's enough. Stop it (pseudo quiet-determination) . . . . Aw, come on, stop it (whine) . . . Well, what do you want me to do? . . . Ow, that hurts (a little whine, but more honest expression of pain) . . . Stop it (a little anger) . . . Shit, stop it! That's enough!! " (Now the anger is true. His face is unmasked, his voice is serious and we continue with his expression of honest rage.)

Tension in the orbital muscles, revealed in the inability to follow movements in the visual field with dexterity, can be corrected by a number of maneuvers. The patient may roll his eyes as quickly as possible in a circle looking around the room at the walls. The object is to attain the maximum speed without the sacrifice of particulate sight. This technique and the several to follow are essentially exercises in concentration and in permitting the eyes to be excited. They are difficult to perform, as is any exercise that demands full concentration.

An alternative maneuver is to have the patient follow random movements of a finger or a flashlight within the visual field. The flashlight is more commonly used in therapy because the photic stimulation of the electric light seems to add to visual excitement. Dr. Barbara Goldenberg Koopman[13] has done fascinating work in this area. In all of these visual motor activities, the therapist is an active participant, concentrating on picking up flagging patient concentration, goading the patient to greater speed and focus. The therapist does not merely set the patient in motion and sit back comfortably to watch the performance.

The inability of some individuals to perform these moving-seeing exercises for more than a few seconds seems astonishing to many. The process reveals the presence of dissociative processes in many people.

[13]Baker, Elsworth F., *Man In The Trap*, The Macmillan Co., N.Y., 1967, pp. 50-52.

"That's strange. I start out determined to really follow the light. I know it's a simple thing to do. But then, I don't know when it happens, I'm suddenly thinking about something altogether different, or else I'm thinking about doing it, instead of actually doing it."

Perceptive patients describe the effort of following a darting object as trying to pull the eyes around against the resistance of strong rubber bands. The continued exertion often results in gradually decreased muscular tension and a new visual clarity.

Over a long period of time, the endeavor to move the eyes and see uncovers frustration and rage. In those yet unable to rage, the frustration may lead to crying. For those patients who early in childhood learned the trick of dealing with life's difficulties by going off in the eyes either into a fantasy reverie or into a state of utter blankness, a mountain of work must be done to unhinge this automatic mechanism. The therapist instructs the patient to go into the eyes-off state voluntarily and then to suddenly pull his eyes back into focused contact. This maneuver requires the utmost concentration in individuals unused to concentrating. It is used in conjunction with the work in eye tracking (following the flashlight or finger with the eyes).

Once patients have discovered their tendency to separate themselves from the environment by going off in their eyes and have learned how the performance of eye movements can help bring them back into contact with their environment, they can use this knowledge when they lose concentration. Students, for example, learn that after hours at their books when they begin to reread each sentence, they must take a brief vacation from the print, and move their eyes quickly round the room, apprehending as many visual details as possible. After several concentrated minutes of this work, they can return to their books and understand each sentence as they read it.

For those who need it, work on eye comprehension is not restricted to the treatment hour. The therapist instructs patients to grasp as much detail as possible as they pass store windows, then return to see what they have missed. The also must pick out such details as color, design, and texture of the clothing of people in the street as well as peculiarities in their gait and facial expressions. To people who have never looked, the emotions on the faces of their fellows always come as a surprise.

From the therapeutic standpoint, these are not merely mechanical exercises. The patient with a large emotional stake in deadened eyes will resist strongly. As the dead eyes learn once again to see, the patient will experience a rise in anxiety, which must be dealt with. Occasionally a strong breakthrough in eye armoring will precipitate acute anxiety, which will need immediate care.

In the course of therapy, the patient with armored eyes must become capable of the expression of all emotions in his eyes. He must be able to look and feel tenderly in his eyes, to look violently angry, terrified, deeply sad. In eliciting these emotions, the therapist interacts with the patient, feeling and expressing these emotions in his own face and eyes.

After many hours of work and fifteen defensive ploys, a patient arrives at the point where she and I are looking at one another openly, warmly, without subterfuge. The patient's face is transfigured; it is not her previous face. She says, "You know I never made a place for love in my life."

A schizophrenic patient who is having great difficulty with eye tenderness says, "When I let my eyes go soft and look at you, I feel as if you're going to come at me and beat me up. When I keep my eyes the usual way I'm not scared of you."

A young man attempting to express eye rage throws his head around as if it were almost independent of his body. I explain that he throws the head about in this fashion to disclaim responsibility for his anger, as if the anger were independent of him. When he attempts to "take charge" of his anger by coordinating head and body, he can no longer express the anger.

A patient succeeds finally in expressing anger with his eyes. His face is flushed, contorted with rage, sneering, bitter. Afterward he says, "I really started to hate you. I felt like tearing your eyes out. How can that happen? Because I really like you."

As another patient lets tenderness through her eyes, she says, "I recognized that I never looked at any men, not even Larry (her mate); and I suddenly wanted to hit you. You became my father, and I knew I was afraid of being seduced. I couldn't look at men because of him."

Working temporarily on another segment, I ask a patient to try to feel the pleasure of breathing down without resistance. The patient tries for a while, then interrupts himself. He says (correctly), "Doc, how can I feel pleasure? I can't even look you in the eyes yet."

One of the most terrifying procedures, especially for individuals with a palpable level of anxiety, is to open the eyes widely, raise the forehead, emphasize the inspiratory phase of respiration (as in actual fright) and permit fear to come into the eyes. If the patient can muster the courage, the experience often precipitates an anxiety attack. And often, in the throes of the fear, the memory of the fearsome events that eventuated in armoring rise to the surface in three-dimensional vision.

Moving the eyes to their lateral limits simulates the suspicious gaze of the paranoid as he looks for signs of danger. This sidelong glance helps make patients more aware of their suspiciousness.

One repeats the same maneuvers time after time in therapy. A patient who experiences a hint of suspicion on one occasion may, at some further point in therapy, feel suspicious to the point of paranoia. Or at one time the patient may experience deep rage in his eyes, but at a later repetition, may come upon a layer of rage more consuming than he thought possible.

In addition to the commonly used techniques for dealing with the armoring of a particular segment, every therapist adds his own variations or borrows from his life experience or his medical knowledge to bring something new to practice.

For example, a patient with severe eye block also complained of chronic pain in one ear. Direct work on the eyes and the affected ear did little to relieve the pain. On one occasion when the patient described the difficulty she was having with reading, transposing letters and syllables, I inquired into her handedness. She said that she was ambidextrous, that she had been born left-handed, but that handedness had been switched in childhood. I instructed her to put a patch over one eye for increasing periods daily and to begin retraining her left hand in writing. Within a week, the ear pain diminished. The problem was not completely solved because the patient still complained that the ear felt "closed" (though her hearing was adequate), but she was relieved of pain.

Eye armoring dissolves to some extent when brain functions are improved through conventional means. When irrational thought gives way to reason or a person attains a deeply experienced insight, the knotted brain clears, bringing more clarity to the eyes. The formerly chaotic, backward patients who with conditioning techniques have learned to eat with utensils without slopping themselves are, to a small degree, less eye-armored for the experience.

One often hears claims about the profound insights that the use of this or that street drug will bestow. The claims are overblown, but certain drugs do seem to have the potential for loosening brain armoring, and in rare instances of bestowing new and valid insights on their users. However, taken all in all, the end result of such drug use is far more harmful than helpful. Armoring released in the eye segment can not be therapeutically useful when it is loosed against an otherwise heavily armored body. As a matter of fact, one often observes that the eye segment is more heavily armored after the effects of smoking marihuana have worn-off. The expansion that follows loosening of brain armoring by the drug is succeeded by a reactive contraction, and the result is a net loss so far as emotional health is concerned. Chaos can result from the clash of grace in a graceless corpus; and these are the drug takers who require hospitalization. In most cases the armored body will gradually smother the enlivened brain, and the individual will continue in his life as dead as ever, with eyes devoid of luminosity.

Deadness in the eye segment often spurs efforts to "get something moving up there," and individuals poke their scalps, rub their eyes, and, in the case of severely armored children, bang their heads.

A patient with eyes sorely out of contact is subjected to my painfully prodding fingers in the parietal area. he says, "I know it hurts, but I don't even feel like yelling. In a way it even feels good. Does that mean that I like to suffer?"

To be free of armoring in the eye segment implies that the mind acts in conjunction with natural emotions and is not used to provide "rational" defenses against them. Unarmored eyes, informed, attain insight. The husband with armored eyes sees his anxious, harried, distraught, coping wife and makes jokes about her behavior. The husband with unarmored eyes sees that she is distracted and that she copes, but he senses the terror from which she flees and he is not jocular.

The Oral Segment
In dealing with the armoring of the oral segment, which involves a considerable part of the facial musculature, the therapist often uses a mirror -- either the actual glass or the mirror of imitation. If the patient is to become aware of his pouty, or angry, or scared, or overbright face, he must see it as we see it. I mold my face as the patient molds his in order to reveal him to himself. Sometimes the anger that his overbright face conceals is elicited as I persist in an imitation. Sometimes he cries childishly, the next step inward, as I pout back his pout.

Patients must learn to express all emotions in their faces. Free breathing aids in providing energy for this task, and sometimes the appropriate uses of other segments, for example, clawing hands or pounding fists (thoracic segment), also help. Emotional involvement is a *sine qua non* in this process; it alone provides authenticity. In patients who have been trained to bland affect, the work is arduous.

A patient, whose face as she lies on the couch is a constant mask with lips slightly pursed and eyes glued to a spot in the ceiling, works on making a pleasant face. For the better part of an hour, she tries and it is all mechanical; but at one point, and for the first time since I have known her, her face eases into a genuine smile. When the session is over, she says, "I feel as if I've been through a wringer."

For the facial muscles to convey an emotion in its full force, the eye segment must be at least partially mobilized, because the expression in the eyes is integral to any meaningful facial expression. Work on the eyes also includes work on the facial muscles; they may be mobilized together.

Two therapeutic maneuvers deal with the anger contained in a tightly held jaw. First, the therapist prods the musculature with his fingers (usually a painful procedure); second, the patient bites as forcefully as possible, feeling his anger as he bites. Where the jaw armoring is chronic and heavy, patients are often instructed to practice biting on cloth or leather at home.

A young woman, whose jaw armoring had been dealt with in the past, and whose therapy had proceeded through the abdominal segment, developed intense rearmoring in the jaw segment, with tooth-gnashing at night and clamping of the jaw by day to the point of pain. She was advised to do lots of towel-biting as homework.

On the following visit she reported, "I've been practicing the biting and one day I suddenly knew what I wanted to hold on to. I was biting my father's finger. I've read enough to know what that means. And then the back of my throat opened, and then muscles on the inside of my thigh that had always been tight before."

When the patient's jaw is armored, the mobility of the mouth -- including the sucking function -- is impaired. To bring back the mobility, the therapist advises thumb-sucking. It is often extremely distasteful to those individuals for whom weaning was a traumatic process, or those who sucked their thumbs and were shamed for it. Some patients have such sensitive lips that they cannot bear having them touched; others cannot put their thumb to their lips without gagging.

As the result of emotional breakthroughs in other segments, one often sees involuntary tremors in the muscles of the mouth and lips. As the tremors develop, they sometimes are revealed as a last ditch effort of the mouth to suppress crying. More often, when the free play of these apparently random twitchings is encouraged, they take shape as infantile sucking movements and are associated with recovery of infantile memories.

Where sucking has been interfered with in childhood, the patient is unable to suck softly with pleasure; the sucking is either mechanical or avaricious. Sometimes, when the patient begins to perceive pleasure in sucking, he almost simultaneously feels pleasure in his pelvis. Often, however, pelvic anxiety will interfere with the patient's freedom to indulge in the oral satisfaction.

The patient, who had sucked her thumb till she was nine and broken herself of the act through rigid self-discipline, lies crying and yelling. Her voice has a childish quality. Suddenly she is quiet and her eyes open wide. She stays this way for several moments, perturbed but absorbed. Her lips begin to move in a distorted sucking pattern, then she sobs in huge heartbroken waves. When she is again quiet I ask, "What did you see?" "A huge breast filled with sour milk," she replies.

The vocal function of the oral segment is to express feelings -- rage, sadness, fear; to yell and scream and cry; and, through the subtle modulations of the voice, to convey the gentler feelings. The therapist works not only on the intensity of the vocal expression but on its quality. Each voice has a natural timbre and range. A sensitive listener can hear any constraint on these natural notes of speech. The whisperers, the bellowers, the whiners -- these are only some of the ways people violate their natural voices.

A big, robust man, who conducts his life so that he's liked by everyone, has a large, resonant voice -- which he rarely uses. In a previous session he sang for me and his voice is glorious. Now he lies on the couch sighing through a squeezed, tight throat and his chin is tense. I direct him to make a bigger, more open sound, but as the volume increases so does the strain.

It seems to me that his reluctance to use his resonant natural voice is related to problems of character. "That big voice commits you," I tell him, "It makes you a target. It's deep and important. It says, 'This is not a nice guy; it's me.' You can use it when you sing because that doesn't commit you; you're only singing. That's probable one of the reasons you enjoy singing so much; you can be your deep, big self without putting yourself on the line. You're like the stutterer; he can sing without stuttering."

The patient replies, "Oh, wow, I'm so fucking good on the stage, and I know it. But if I spoke like that in a bar, somebody might pick a fight."

The natural quality of the voice cannot come through until the emotions entrapped in the armored musculature -- for example, the crying or the screaming -- have been released. It is not simply a matter of vocal training. In some cases the emotion cannot be released until the throat has been loosened in gagging. The therapist threads his way from emotional block to emotional block.

A patient attempting to scream is obviously going through a traumatic experience. Her expression has the quality of a tantrum. She stops and breathes for a while, then goes into the screaming again, but this time the performance is much wilder and piercing. When it is over she asks, "You want to know what happened?" She says, "The first time I was having a tantrum on the street when I was a little girl walking with my parents. That actually happened. The second time I decided to make it come out better and I was yelling so loud that I'd attract the attention of a policeman and he'd come and take me away from my parents. That never happened but I wish it had."

The muscles under the chin are often instrumental in holding crying; and just as one watches for swallowing as a way patients keep from crying, one keeps an eye on the submental muscles (the muscles under the chin). When they are taut, the therapist subjects them to painful finger pressure until the patient's cry is released.

A section on the voice in therapy would be incomplete without a word on the patients' verbal communications. So much of human expression is a flight from feeling, thinking or saying something of import. As armoring in the eye segment converts the brain from an organ that intelligently solves the body's problems to one that rationalizes why it should continue to perform in its crippled fashion, armoring in the oral segment acts as the verbal courier of the "cockeyed" brain. Consequently, it is not uncommon at the end of a patient's recitation for the therapist to comment, "Bullshit!" One does not permit the patient to crowd the treatment room with verbal garbage any more than one permits his defensive smile to go unchallenged. Patients who are masters at verbal defense are made to shut up. On the other hand, thoughtful, deeply felt discussions are welcomed in their appropriate time. For it is true: thoughtful words are as important in conveying deep feeling as more dramatic expressions such as crying and screaming.

The patient, a man in his early forties, raised in a fundamentalist church, is requested to yell the vilest, most obscene words at the top of his voice. After repeated refusals he consents, beginning with "shucks" and "darn" and upwards to expressions that would be credible in a navy barracks. But he is only saying, not shouting them. I urge him to scream them at the top of his lungs. He finally does, and they come pouring forth with affect. He stops suddenly. His eyes are raised apprehensively to the ceiling. He is waiting for God's thunderbolt.

Certain aspects of oral armoring are treated as problems of character as well as physical problems. The most dependent persons, for example, make their way through life looking for sustaining nipples. In therapy this would be worked through on both the behavioral and physical levels.

The Cervical Segment

Treatment of armoring in the cervical segment involves handling problems of the lower reaches of the throat, the deep cervical musculature and the superficial posterior cervical musculature as well as further work on gagging. Ordinarily most of the painfully taut cervical muscles lie in the posterolateral and posterior area of the neck.

Crying, screaming, yelling, raging and tender sighing are elicited to enable the patient to express whatever emotions have been problematic. It is interesting that on occasion the repeated utterance of deep, satisfied "ahh" sounds with a fully opened throat eliminates the wheeze in an asthmatic attack of mild to moderate severity.

The therapist deals with stubbornness on both a characterological and physical level. The stubborn muscles lie posteriorly, and he attacks them by painful pressure, which evokes the rage that lies behind the stubborn defiance. To become acquainted with the muscles of stubbornness, patients are requested to stiffen their necks and experience the resistance in its fullness. Later they are encouraged to shake their heads from side to side while yelling words like, "No" or "I won't." Sometimes the forcible dorsi-flexion of the neck to a point where the mouth lies in a plane with the throat succeeds in releasing deep sobbing held back by a tight ring of cervical armoring.

In those individuals in whom cervical armoring represents the fear of being struck, the emphasis is on the expression of the fear, then the fury in reaction.

To counter the stiffness in motion and the anxiety that free-wheeling neck movements engender in those with cervical armoring, patients perform free-swinging neck, shoulder and arm movements as in dancing. The anxiety that such loose cervical motion elicits is often surprising in its intensity. To those unaware of the general fear of surrender in the neck it would be instructive to perform the following experiment: Lift a baby by supporting him between the shoulders or by taking both of his arms. The healthy infant will permit his back to be raised without resistance; and as his chest rises, his head and neck fall backward gracefully. Now repeat the same maneuver with adults. Note how in most cases the head and neck rise rigidly as the chest is raised. To surrender in one's neck is to be undefended -- a dangerous posture in a hostile world.

The Thoracic Segment

In working on thoracic armoring, the therapist looks at the area's functions. There is the breathing activity, which not only sustains life but regulates the energy level of the body. Then there is the aggressive and defensive function of the upper limbs, the surrender of the lower chest bordering on the diaphragm, the holding-back function of the dorsal spinal region, the protective function of shoulders turtled to cover the neck, and the longing for union of outstretched arms.

The therapist encourages deep breathing and keeps an eye out lest the patient's respiration decline. Sometimes he tells patients to place their hands on their chests to become more aware of chest movement in breathing. Sometimes the therapist places his hands over the patient's sternum and pushes forcefully with each expiration until his chest begins to move spontaneously.

Despite this forced aid, sometimes the chest will not move until one has dealt with the armored intercostal muscles. In the axillary or lower rib or dorsal area the therapist applies pressure, which may get at held emotions and enable the chest to move freely. Where there is muscular hypersensitivity, tickling may have the same effect, or sometimes the softest stroking over the hypersensitive area will work.

Just as there is a natural timbre and range for each voice, there is a natural respiratory rate above which the organism is energized and below which it merely maintains life functions. Patients unconsciously discover that when they breathe at a certain rate, nothing frightening will happen; and they attempt to hold their breathing to this rate. The therapist must be aware of this fact and encourage them to breathe faster. In contrast, some patients huff like a steam engine in the attempt to precipitate some dramatic effect. This unnatural mechanical exercise must also be discouraged.

In encouraging breathing, the therapist must be aware of the patient's general energetic status and tolerance. In an organism tight to the bursting point, a sudden increase in energy generated in the chest could conceivably precipitate a psychotic episode or a cardiac accident.

A bright, energetic, relatively new young patient lies breathing, savoring the experience. I caution her to slow down, but she reassures me that this experience is too pleasant to diminish. As she continues, it is apparent that she is becoming uncomfortable; and just at the point where I decide to tell her to stop all activity, she begins to scream. The screaming goes on for minutes; her pupils are saucer-wide and her palms drenched with cold sweat. I cuddle her and the screams subside gradually. She is all atremble and continues in soft moans. Later, when she has recovered she says, "It just happened suddenly, I got scared and I thought I was going crazy."

Patients express the aggressive uses of the upper extremities in a variety of ways. They pound on a couch and occasionally on the rug-covered wall (though the latter is not encouraged). In punching, it is important that the patient put his entire force into the blow, that no energy be lost in the play of inhibitory muscles, and that strong emotion accompany the effort. Females are permitted to punch the therapist's arm in the padded deltoid area unless it begins to hurt. Sometime a sheet is shaped into head size and patients visualize the face of their momentary enemy as they pound.

A patient's impulse to throttle is gratified by encircling the therapist's forearm and squeezing with all his might. Scratching and pinching are vented on the couch mattress. Occasionally patients are granted the pleasure of ripping the sheet to shreds.

The importance of the muscular discharge of energy through the hands is attested to by many natural phenomena, the tremor of the outstretched hands of the anxiety -- ridden, the pan-cultural habit of wringing hands, drumming fingers, rubbing fingers, counting beads for distraction. However, in encouraging the physical release of rage, the therapist must know his patient. Where there is doubt about ego control, one moves slowly. And, as in all of the rest of life, sometimes one takes calculated risks.

A meek and mild borderline psychotic in her early thirties has been working on the repressed aggression in her shoulders and arms. Throughout therapy she has been voicing dissatisfaction with her husband to whom she is tied in a dependency-hate relationship. He has been the target of all her hostile outpourings. On the day her rage finally erupts in therapy, she is seized with reactive anxiety and she says that she fears that now she might kill her husband. I reassure her that she has sufficient control to keep from doing such a thing.

In the middle of the night I am awakened by a phone call. The patient is on the line and she says that after her husband fell asleep she arose from bed, went to the kitchen, returned with a knife and cut his wrist. Then she woke him, told him what she had done and bandaged his wound. I ask to speak to the husband. When he came to the phone, he could hardly speak for laughing. "The nick is so small," he said, "I don't see how it could have bled at all."

The symbolic murder marked a turning point in the therapy and in the marital relationship.

The process of releasing shoulder girdle hostility is speeded up when the patient simultaneously makes hateful eye contact. This is the time when patients recognize that they harbor murderous impulses toward the therapist -- impulses which had been hidden from consciousness. Patients are often at a loss to account for the fact that they wish to kill, or at least hurt, someone who has been helpful and considerate. The therapist explains at this point that he represents humanity, that the rage is not against his person but against what he represents.

In several decades of practice, only one patient made me apprehensive for my safety. He was a huge hulk of a man who once in a bar room brawl had beaten-up his adversary and then turned the juke-box over his fallen foe.

Patients who learn to express their rage in therapy do not go about thereafter beating up their families, friends and neighbors. They are less prone to suffer aggression passively, and they tend to function more aggressively (but not hostilely) in all aspects of their lives. In my experience there was one brief exception to this generalization.

A patient had rioted and raged for the first time on the couch; and having been submissive for most of his life, he relished the experience and left the session in high spirits. On the next visit, he told the following story:

"When I left your office," he said, "I was feeling wonderful. And as I walked toward the subway station I had the feeling that I wanted to get into a fight. When I was a kid I used to run away from fights, and when I got to the subway station the impulse was really strong. I started talking to some dude on the platform, and I knew that I was deliberately taunting him. Well, finally he had a neckful of me and we got into it. I gave him a couple of good ones and knocked him down. Then I helped him to get up and apologized to him and told him he could give me a couple, but he didn't want to. He must have thought I was out of my mind."

A variant technique for bringing out upper extremity aggression is for the therapist to pin the patient's arms to the couch above his head and tell the patient to throw the therapist off and free his arms using any means except biting. Both the weak, hopeless struggles of some patients and the energetic battles of others are a gauge of the aggressive energies of the patient. The dispatch with which some thin muscled ladies can unburden themselves of the therapist's oppression attests to the power of focused energy and purpose.

To elicit the tender uses of the upper extremities, the therapist tells the patient to reach with outstretched arms while sighing with longing. Because of the cultural mold, this is particularly difficult for many men to do. It flies in the face of the "macho" model in which little boys have often been set. Consequently, it is males who often have the strongest emotional breakthroughs in the performance of this act.

The patient practices the soft-touching uses of his hands by enclosing the therapist's hand in his, perceiving warm tactile contact. Or the patient may touch the therapist's face, maintaining warm eye contact. Tender touching suffers from the same cultural abnegation as reaching out. It is instructive in watching films of the stone-age Tasaday in the Philippines or of premodern Eskimos to see how much communication is transmitted by touch in those less-armored societies.

I ask a wooden patient to hold my hand in hers. She cannot bear to close her fingers around my hand; and when she finally does, she must close her eyes.

The patient whose shoulders rise in defense of the neck must learn, particularly in times of stress, to proceed with loose, lowered shoulders. The aggressive and defensive uses of the shoulder girdle have a reciprocal relationship. The more the individual becomes capable of aggressive action, the less tendency he has to automatic defense, and the less the shoulders rise.

The therapist treats spite that is held in tightened bands of paraspinal muscles between the scapulae with firm, probing pressure that releases the rage that lies under the spite.

The Diaphragmatic Segment

The therapist's work on the diaphragmatic armoring aims at destroying the impedance function of the armored diaphragm so that impulses of excitation can proceed through this area unhindered. The practice of gagging while breathing in and out freely is one of the chief techniques employed. Patients with a strong diaphragmatic block are encouraged to gag upon arising. Another mechanical aid is to have the patient practice the movement and sound of "belly" laughter or convulsive sobbing, assuming that whatever blocks might have existed in the throat have been eradicated. Or the therapist tickles the hypersensitive muscles in the diaphragmatic region, taking care that the laughter is released freely and openly.

When the therapist has succeeded in relieving the diaphragmatic block, permitting the patient to breathe through, the greatest barrier between pleasurable impulse source and the target genital excitation has often been removed. Consequently, patients sometimes experience a surge of sexual fantasy and sexual dream material at this point. Or, if the pelvis is almost totally blocked, the diaphragmatic breakthrough may appear as violent rage.

In the preceding week's session the patient had succeeded in breathing through for the first time. At his next session he told the following story: "Last Wednesday I was trying to breathe and let my chest go and suddenly the same thing happened that happened here last week, and everything seemed to melt all the way down to my pelvis. Then I went into a fantasy: it just came over me that I was having intercourse with my mother. Then I remembered that when I was about thirteen I dreamed that I was having intercourse with my mother and that was the last wet dream I ever had. But when I woke from that dream I felt so miserable and guilty that I couldn't stand it. I guess that's why I didn't think about it till this happened."

When the diaphragmatic block has been removed, the patient can gag and vomit easily. At this point a physical wave runs down the abdomen, which the patient may observe as well as perceive subjectively.

The Abdominal Segment

The dissolution of abdominal armoring is usually a fairly straightforward matter. One of the therapist's commonest techniques is to press a finger in the midline between the xiphoid process and the umbilicus (the belly button). Each time the patient breathes out, the therapist presses fairly gently, and this pressure often softens the taut musculature sufficiently to permit the abdominal wave to proceed. In other cases, more severe pressure laterally along the margins of the rectus abdominis is necessary. Occasionally, after the therapist has relaxed the musculature in the upper abdomen, there is a residue of tension in the low abdomen, especially above the pubic area. Pressure here releases spite that is held in the armored lumbar muscles. It is sometimes advantageous for the patient to bang his belly against the couch repeatedly to get at abdominal rage.

Reich indicates in his writing that when one has freed armoring above the abdominal segment, the work on the abdomen proceeds easily. In my experience, this has often been so, but there have also been instances where the progress of therapy has been held up for months at the abdominal segment. It may be that in this latter case the abdominal armoring represents the last line of defense for a not-too-heavily armored pelvis.

After months of consistent attack, the abdominal armoring of a young male patient finally gave way. Spontaneously, he remarked on how tense his arms and buttocks felt at this point. When he voluntarily relaxed them, he found himself walking in a new way. These events that occurred in the pelvic segment were almost like a follow-through to the dissolution of the abdominal armoring.

The Pelvic Segment

The patient with an armored pelvis who attempts to move his pelvis usually moves thighs, pelvis and abdomen in one piece. Independent pelvic movement is difficult when the muscles in and around the pelvis are tense.

The regions that tend to greatest tension are the pelvic floor, the buttocks and perianal area, the thigh adductors and the posterior thigh musculature.

Work on the armoring in the pelvic segment precipitates more anxiety than work on other segments. No anxiety is so deep as this anxiety. For this reason work on the pelvic armoring is left for the last in therapy. Only when the armoring in all other segments has been dealt with and the organism has gained a certain solidity does one embark on treating the pelvic segment. And one proceeds cautiously.

The simple act of breathing down and permitting the thighs to open gently on respiratory expiration is sufficient to occasion anxiety in some patients, especially female.

A young woman who had performed this simple exercise for the first time in her therapy session reported at her next visit: "I knew when I was doing it that it was upsetting me, but I didn't know how much. Every night last week I had dreams of horrible punishment and it got to the point where I was afraid to go to sleep. All that from opening my legs a little bit."

Another patient performing the same exercise says, "I have to keep telling myself that I'm not trying to seduce my father, and I'm afraid of what will happen when that wall comes down."

The almost universal armoring of the adductors of the thighs is observed as the patient lies breathing with her thighs apart. In some there is an observable periodic spasm as the thighs fight to close together, in others the armoring is only recognized upon palpation of the taut adductors. Reich facetiously dubbed these adductors the "morality muscles." The therapist treats both the superficial and deep adductors by painful pressure both on the muscular belly and above their point of insertion. The pain increases the patient's awareness of the armoring and often elicits the story of the affect buried in the armoring. The same procedures are employed in dealing with the posterior thigh muscles, chiefly the biceps femoris (the largest of the hamstring muscles).

After the armoring of the thigh musculature has been dealt with, one proceeds to the tension in the sacral and buttock areas. The patient is made aware of the tension in the buttocks by voluntarily tightening and releasing this musculature; here, too, the therapist applies painful pressure to these taut muscles.

One then treats the tension of the anal sphincters by instructing the patient to tighten the sphincters with inspiration and to let them go with expiration. An alternative is to instruct the patient to tighten the sphincters and to maintain the tension for as long as possible while breathing.

A patient reports: "You know I noticed that every time I put my foot on the brake I tighten my anus. Now that's really weird. That must mean that anytime I want to stop anything I automatically tighten my ass."

Once patients have mastered the armoring about the anal sphincter, they frequently report a change in bowel habits. Disorders such as constipation usually disappear and the patients experience a new pleasure in bowel functions.

In order to deal with the pelvic armoring, the patient must first perceive that it is there. Sometimes patients are completely unaware that a muscle group is held in a state of constant contraction; this is most true of the muscles of the pelvic floor. Often, as the patient breathes, the scrotum can be observed to rise with each breath, as the pelvic floor muscles contract; yet the patient assumes he is totally relaxed. There is no comparable external sign for the females. To apprise the patient of this contraction, the therapist instructs him to voluntarily contract the pelvic floor musculature for as long as he can possibly hold it, then to let go. For the first time he recognizes what relaxed musculature in this area feels like. An alternative method is to instruct the patient to tighten the muscles with inspiration and to relax them with expiration. Then he is instructed to be aware of the contraction or relaxation of these muscles as he proceeds with his activities during the week.

When some of the armoring has been loosened, the patient is in a position to practice the voluntary movement of the pelvis with breathing. The pelvis must move independently of thighs and abdomen, and it is here that acute anxiety is often experienced. At this juncture in therapy patients who had enjoyed a satisfying sex life often report cessation of all sexual desire, or a sudden difficulty with sexual performance -- frigidity, impotence, anesthesia -- that had never occurred before. This difficulty is always temporary and coincides with the new layer of sexual anxiety that has been plumbed. Once this difficulty is passed, the sexual experience rises to new, and heretofore unexperienced heights.

The voluntary pelvic movement is not designed as practice for sexual performance but as a means of eradicating the pelvic stiffness which prohibits the appearance of involuntary pelvic movement, the orgasm reflex.

The appearance of the orgasm reflex always comes as a surprise to the patient the first time it occurs. One patient said, "It feels like a magnet making your pelvis move, and you have nothing to do with it." In the beginning it is always experienced with at least a modicum of anxiety, no matter how much sexual anxiety has already been cleared.

With the elimination of armoring an awareness of the connection of the pelvic segment with the rest of the body develops.

While the work is proceeding on the pelvic armoring, patients report new sensations perceived in the genital area. Females describe warmth, tingling, and melting sensations deep in the vagina; males report similar feelings in the penis, often accompanied by erections. With time, the sensations perceived in the therapeutic hour become incorporated in the sexual performance at home. Generally, the patient is several years out of therapy by the time new sexual freedom is totally integrated into his sex life.

A final note: Because of the damage we see being wrought on patients in "neo-Reichian" therapies, we must reemphasize this warning: The pelvic segment must be approached only after armoring has been cleared in upper segments. When the pelvic segment is approached prematurely, the body attempts to deal with the overwhelming anxiety by increasing the blocking at higher levels. Sometimes this last ditch, desperate attempt to hold back energy from reaching the pelvis creates armoring of such intensity that it is no longer amenable to therapeutic efforts.

Chapter 6
The Theory of Orgone Energy

A middle-aged man recently developed a fear of going over bridges -- a fear that greatly interferes with his work. For several months preceding the onset of the phobia, he had been thinking that he might harm his wife, even though he said that she gave him absolutely no cause for such hostility; and he had become uneasy in the presence of sharp kitchen knives. He had been raised in a strict, patriarchal household and admitted that he might feel some hostility toward his father.

How shall we view this development of a phobia? Having elicited this history, the analytically oriented psychiatrist would recognize the classic lines of development. Hostility was repressed in infancy and childhood. An equilibrium was established between the repressing forces and the repressed affect that held pretty well until several months preceding the emergence of the bridge phobia. (The psychiatrist is aware that a more complete history will reveal many other signs of disequilibrium along the way, but none of sufficient intensity to cause the patient to seek help.) Then, for a reason yet to be determined, the repression cracked; the affect broke through in the guise of thoughts about hurting his wife. After several months this new equilibrium failed. The anxiety level was rising and was now placed on an innocuous object in the environment -- the bridge.

The analyst's plan is clear. The patient must learn to face the anxiety that his repressed childhood rage incurs. His insight into the problem will help him in this task and, to the extent that he expresses his anger in his therapeutic sessions and in his social relationships, the anxiety will decrease. This is the bare bones of the therapeutic effort. In a long-term analysis, other material will be uncovered, and the relationship of the patient to therapist will be explored; but this is not pertinent to the present discussion. The essence of the matter is that the analyst will explore unconscious psychological processes with the patient. If the psychiatrist is competent and the patient cooperative, the intensity of the phobic reaction will decrease or, perhaps, disappear.

The behaviorist takes a different view of the situation. To him the symptom is a learned response, the product of faulty conditioning. His therapeutic endeavor will be aimed at behavior modification. He will set up procedures to desensitize the patient. Using either aversion training (suffering for doing the wrong thing) or rewards for right performance, he will condition his patient to cross bridges. If the therapist is competent and the program sound, the patient may be enabled to cross bridges.

Though the theoretical bases of the psychoanalyst and the behaviorist are disparate, they both function within the framework of psychology. In this, they differ from the orgonomic view.

The orgonomist assesses the patient with a phobic reaction and he sees -- a disturbance of biological pulsation. The psychoanalyst focuses on the unconscious and its manifestations, the behaviorist on the symptom, the orgonomist on the energy economy of the patient's organism.

Whatever the disorder, be it somatic or psychological (with only few exceptions such as parasitic infestation, accidents, congenital defects), the orgonomist seeks for the root of the disease in an aberration of energy metabolism. In the case of a phobia, the therapist might treat the symptom by encouraging his patient to face his fear, but he would not expect any radical symptomatic improvement until some alteration in the disturbed energy flow had been effected. He would treat all symptoms -- from ulcers to impotence to psychosis -- the same way. Not that he would delay the surgical excision of an acutely inflamed appendix while he attempts to remove the abdominal armoring. We are talking of sources and origins. Some disease processes that arise because of disturbance of energy flow progress to a point where they can no longer be dealt with by altering source mechanisms. They must then be treated by conventional medical means.

As physician, the orgonomist is philosophically opposed to the tendency of twentieth-century medicine to become more specialized. Though he admires the technical achievement of modern medicine, such as cardiac surgery and replacement therapy, he decries the search for thousands of new varieties of drugs with which to treat hundreds of symptoms. He decries the blindness which never sees the crucial disordered biological functioning that generates symptoms in profusion. With his conventional colleagues, he welcomes the discovery of effective antibiotics with which to combat infections; but unlike them, the orgonomist is aware that an energetically blocked organism is prone to succumb to infections. Like them, he is aware of the potential carcinogenic effects of cigarettes, air pollutants, food additives and nuclear radiation; but unlike them, he sees that characterologic resignation provides a more fertile soil in which these irritants can work their damage. The orgonomist is the spiritual brother to the engineer who is obsessed with preparing measures to keep the river flowing in its bed at flood tide, not to the engineer who engages in heroics as the river floods its banks.

Orgonomists are in a unique position to observe the pulses of orgone energy in the human organism. As students and physicians, we observe the pulses of the organ systems -- the throb of the heart, the beat of the respiratory apparatus, the rhythm of the peristaltic wave, the beat in the exposed brain and the occasionally observed crawling pulse of the scrotum. From Reich we learn of the wandering-forth beat of the peripheral nerves and the end receptors.

We watch as our patients, after breaking through an armoring block, are seized with a wave of rage or crying or tenderness; then it subsides and they are at ease. Slowly the emotion builds to another peak and subsides again. It may build to a climax after its original release, or the first release may be the deepest and it gradually declines. But always there are the pulse, the beats, the tides. When the patient is alive and free of encumbrance, the therapist is observer to the heart of Nature.

At these moments the patients are aware that they are the vessels of the emotions they express. At no time is the validity of Reich's insight -- that we are veins of energy in a cosmic energy ocean -- so clear as when we are seized by our deepest emotions. Graphically we represent the movement of orgone energy as :

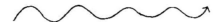

Or in another graphic scheme, Kreiselwelle (the spinning wave form):

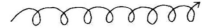

Reich referred to the spinning wave form (known in German as Kreiselwelle) as the movement of orgone energy through time. Through the experience of the pulsation of our emotional expression, we become alive to the curve of the energy; we see its manifestations in every aspect of life. We recognize its flow in the twisting architecture of the long bones in our body, in the spiral path a flower pursues as it grows through the earth, in the energetic bloom and wane as we move from birth to death, in the path our planet winds as it moves through space and time, in the rise and fall of empires, in the vacillation of attitudes toward behavioral issues, in light and dark, life and death. The movement of orgone energy is at the bottom of everything that exists.

A thorough discussion of the experimental work with orgone energy is beyond the scope of this book. Readers with scientific interest in the research on orgone energy are referred to Reich's works and reports from Oranur Laboratories printed in the Journal of Orgonomy, and more recently in the 'Annals of the Institute for Orgonomic Science'.

The psychiatric orgone therapist must keep the following physical properties of orgone energy in mind in performance of his work with patients: Oxygen and water are the basic carriers of orgone energy, so far as living organisms are concerned. Orgone energy is metabolized from the air we breathe, from our food and water, and from our exposure to the atmosphere. Metabolized orgone energy is expelled from the body in the carbon dioxide that we exhale, in the nitrogenous wastes in the urine, in feces, in sweat and expelled gas. In sickness, the dead, metabolized orgone energy tends to increase in the body tissues.

Because of his energetic bias in viewing human activities, the orgonomist uses a vocabulary that is unique in medicine or psychiatry. He views his patients in terms of expansion and contraction, high or low charge. He is aware that when his patient achieves a state of unusual expansiveness, a contraction will surely follow. He recognizes that each individual makes his way through life with an energy range that is constant, possibly a genetic endowment, and that whatever improvement occurs in therapy will take place within the framework of this energy quantum. This does not, of course, imply that a patient in the throes of depression, where available energies are bound and stilled, is destined to pursue the rest of his life in that low energy state, nor that a densely armored patient will not have more vitality when his armoring is dissolved.

The orgonomist regards expansion and contraction in his patients not as a metaphorical description of "feeling good" or "feeling bad," but as concrete physical phenomena. He believes that there is a natural, biological antithesis between pleasure and anxiety. In the former state, energy flows from the core of the organism to the skin surface; this flow toward the periphery brings the ebullience, flushing and warmth that are experienced as pleasure. In anxiety, on the other hand, an energetic drain toward the interior of the body leaves the body surface cold and pallid. The energy withdrawn from the muscles restricts the individual's freedom of movement; that withdrawn from the brain's cortex freezes his thinking to his fear. Others see this as an absence of substantiality and a fearsome incapability to cope. In expansion and contraction the energy impulse is regarded as primary, the physiological and psychological manifestations are secondary. The physiological manifestations are mediated by the vegetative (autonomic nervous system) and the chemical nerve-ending reactions which lead to the effects of blood flow and chemical changes in the tissues. The psychological manifestations are the way that the human being experiences these events.

All emotions are viewed as varieties within the schema of expansion and contraction, as specific configurations of energetic movement and expression. The expression of rage is the energetic flow to, and activation of, the voluntary musculature. In longing, the flow of energy is outward, as in pleasure. Sexual longing is an energetic effluence to the lips, skin and genitals (in anticipation of sexual contact with a loved one) and to the chest and upper extremities, creating the desire to embrace. Insofar as the longing for contact with the loved one is unattainable, the continued flow toward the surface is inhibited; and the emotion, a combination of outward flow and frustration, attains its bittersweet quality. Longing that is non-sexual and is directed toward the completion of one's union with nature is comprised only of the flow toward the chest and arms. It must always remain unsatisfied (with the possible exception of the moment of scientific discovery or artistic creation, when it is converted to the "Eureka!" experience. For a moment the Universe is grasped).

True sadness, which is the experience of frustration or loss, consists of an initial impulse of reaching-out, as in longing, followed by a strong contraction back into oneself. Because of its basic contractive quality, those who experience it tend to withdraw from outside stimuli. Contrariwise, in the attempt to escape from sadness, we try to enlist the aid of a comforting figure toward whom our energies can slowly move and so free ourselves from our sadness. The response to pain inflicted from a source against which we are powerless is sometimes called sadness, but it is not; it is hurt. The common denominator of these two emotional expressions is crying, which in both instances informs those about us that we hurt. The crying of the response to pain has less of the contractive quality than the crying of sadness; also, to some extent, pain usually is accompanied by the vocal expression of anger.

Depression must be distinguished from sadness; it is not truly an emotion if we define emotion as an outward movement of energy or feeling (e-mote). Depression is a state in which energy is contained, rather than in motion. It comes about when hostility cannot be expressed because of characterologic inhibitions and is instead swallowed and turned inward against oneself.

Reich describes the phenomenon of superimposition, for which we have two examples: that of the infant and the maternal breast and that of the interpenetration of the genitals in the sexual embrace. Reich described the phenomenon of superimposition as a full bioenergetic contact of two orgonotic streams, resulting in fusion in a manner specific to natural function.

Regarding breast-feeding, on the deepest level, it is a fusion of the energy flow of infant and mother. The nipple rises toward the tiny mouth as the lips stretch toward the nipple. This process transforms both mother and child. The mother is suffused with the pleasure in her bosom and her delight in the baby; the child with the flow from its embracing mother. The occasional "oral orgasm," the involuntary twitchy muscular discharge of the sucking infant's mouth, is the same basic energetic function on this infantile level as will later occur in the genital embrace. Thus, the orgonomist does not view breast-feeding simply as a way of meeting the child's need for nutrition, nor even as the means of satisfying the infant's oral need (though it certainly does both of these things).

Regarding the sexual embrace, the orgonomist sees the functions ordinarily associated with it -- procreation and pleasure-seeking -- as secondary to the basic function of the fusion of two energy streams and the discharge of accumulated energy.

The discharge function of the orgasm is the keystone upon which the theoretical framework of psychiatric orgone therapy rests. In the course of therapy, as the individual armor rings are successively dealt with and dissolved from the head end downward, a wave appears through the diaphragmatic segment when the armoring has been freed. The wave can be observed by the therapist and perceived by the subject. Often at this time a reflex flexion of the trunk (the head and upper body spontaneously move toward the pelvis) at the end of expiration makes its initial appearance. Since this reflex flexion of the trunk occurs only when there is no significant armoring above the diaphragm, it is obvious that there is a reciprocal relationship between appearance of the flexion reflex and absence of armoring; or, stated positively, the free flow of energy above the diaphragm gives rise, under certain circumstances, to reflex flexion of the trunk.

As the armoring dissolves in the abdominal and pelvic segments, movement develops in the pelvis -- the pelvis flexes toward the trunk at the end of expiration. This reflex approximation of the upper and lower ends of the body is the orgasm reflex. Its full appearance depends upon the absence of armoring throughout the body and a state of pleasurable excitement.

This brief, convulsive spasm is a key to unlocking a vast chamber of understanding. When the armoring is attacked and repressed emotion is released, we understand that the armoring binds emotions that we dare not express. The appearance of an energetic wave through the abdomen after the upper segments have been cleared shows us further that when emotions are released, free-flowing energy is released as well. When one considers that the orgasm reflex appears only when all armoring has been eliminated, and also how fiercely the armoring of the lower segments resists the release of the reflex, we realize that in addition to binding emotion, armoring also binds the energy that would become the orgasm reflex.

When we arrive at this point, we face the question, "Why is the orgasm reflex so perilous that our bodies defend against it with all their force?" To answer this question, we must pose an even more fundamental one: "Why does the orgasm exist, and what is its basic function?"

Obviously the orgasm is an involuntary contraction. In this respect it resembles the pulsation of the jellyfish and the beating heart. In a regularly contracting heart, the contraction occurs at a point following auricular (the upper chambers of the heart) filling. The mechanical tension of the dilated auricles builds to a point at which the blood is discharged into the ventricles (the lower chambers of the heart) and an action (electrical) current is transmitted to the apex (the tip of the heart). The heart then relaxes and is available to refill with blood. The process can be delineated: swelling -- charge -- discharge -- relaxation. The same function pervades all of the hollow organs (Reich called them living bladders). The filling of the bladder with urine leads to bladder contraction and urinary discharge; the filling of the intestine with food bulk leads to the propulsion of the bolus (the food bulk) and the peristaltic wave. This manner of functioning is regarded in orgonomy as a quality of the living organ. The organ does not contract in order to propel the blood, or push the food, or empty the bladder; it contracts because living bladders function according to a basic life formula: tension -- charge -- discharge -- relaxation; that is, the energetic function underlies whatever utilitarian purpose comes to be served. This pulsatory quality provides us with a model for understanding the orgasm reflex and is inherent in all living things.

We must first make clear that orgasm in the orgonomic sense does not consist merely in the ability to reach some type of sexual climax. Orgasm in the orgonomic sense is experienced not just in the genitals but involves body-wide sensations of energetic streaming and the appearance of the orgasm reflex during the genital embrace. The orgasm reflex is the condition in which the body, functioning as a whole, acts specifically to discharge pent-up energies; therefore, the free orgasm is the most complete avenue of energetic discharge. There are other ways of releasing energy -- physical work and productive thought; and there are mechanisms for localized discharge from specific organs -- urination, to relieve the tension in the bladder, defecation for rectal discharge, menstruation and parturition to relieve the swollen, tense uterus. The genuine expression of emotion is an energetic discharge. If there are no inhibitions to their discharge, all of these activities, are experienced as pleasurable. (The occurrence of dysmenorrhea [menstrual cramps] and painful childbirth are not exceptions to this statement if one considers first, that inhibitions are responsible for much of the pain and second, that the ultimate evacuation of the uterus is experienced with relief.) The pleasure, however, derives from the relief of physical tension and energetic discharge, not the other way around.

If total energetic discharge is the function of the orgasm, and if discharge is generally experienced as pleasure, why is there such a mighty opposition and inhibition to its occurrence?

To understand the intensity of the forces arrayed against full, free orgastic discharge we must keep in mind the reciprocity between charge and discharge. It is possible for an orgasm diagramatically represented in the spherical shape to alternate in pulsation as in (a).

a.

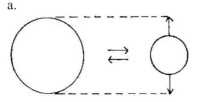

or, b.

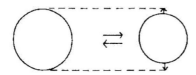

In the first case (a) the circle gets considerably smaller with the contraction phase, so the organism is pulsating maximally. In the second case (b) the circle is only a little smaller in the contraction phase, so the pulsation of the organism is smaller; the range of expansion and contraction is smaller. In example (b) the charge is smaller; and the discharge, represented by the circle becoming only a little smaller, is also less.

The amount of charge depends on the amplitude of discharge and vice versa. Theoretically, a complete discharge suggests that the person is capable of, and will again build, a full charge. In real terms, full charge portends complete emotional ability, openness, sensitivity, vivacity and nothing is more frightening to constrained human beings. So we fight with all our might -- and all our armoring -- to keep the pulse of our lives within bounds that are tolerable. In this culture the spontaneously occurring orgasm reflex is very rarely met, and releasing it in therapy is usually an extensive and toilsome task.

Reich evolved the theory of the function of the orgasm and the orgasm formula (tension-charge-discharge-relaxation) out of his clinical experience. To substantiate its validity and determine whether there were, indeed, measurable energies involved in the experience of pleasure, anxiety and emotional expression, he set up a series of what he called bioelectrical experiments. The work was conducted over a period of several years. Reich measured the electrical potential of the skin in normal people. The skin acts as a porous membrane and carries an electrical potential (the amount of electricity contained in that spot) relative to an area of the skin which has been scraped. He found that all areas of the body except the erogenous zones (and interestingly, the forehead) have a baseline electrical potential which he represented as a horizontal line. The erogenous zones, on the other hand, are characterized by constant variation of the electrical potential, an effect Reich called "wandering." The more emotionally free the subject, the more the tendency to wandering potentials in the erogenous zones. With emotionally rigid subjects, the baseline and erogenous potentials tend not to deviate much from each other.

Pleasurable stimulation of an erogenous area, say, a nipple, results in engorgement of the area stimulated (such as nipple erection) and an increase in electrical potential. However, if the nipple (or other erogenous zone) is stimulated in an irritating manner, what results is a mechanical engorgement of the nipple but a decrease of electrical potential and the experience of displeasure rather than pleasure. The experiments illustrate that mechanical congestion (engorgement) alone cannot lead to energetic charge; in addition, only when congestion is accompanied by a rising orgonotic charge, measured as an increase in electrical potential, is pleasure experienced. Pressure, anxiety and displeasure regularly lead to lowered charge (charge below the normal baseline).

The fact that only with pleasure is there a rise in energy potential and that the rise occurs only at erogenous zones is a statement that sexual pleasure is the stuff of life's productive energy. This is not to be mistaken as a call to a life of untrammeled hedonism. What it says is that only when one is sexually free can the full potential to experience, produce, react, be exercised. To be sexually free is to be alive in the widest sense, and this implies that one also feels sorrow and pain most keenly.

The Nature of Human Nature

Two little Chassidic boys walk in the street in the lower East side of Manhattan. Their pale, denatured faces, their proper gait tell how they have been tamed. Only the life of their intellect and a message of animal sadness speaks in their eyes.

Spiritual cousins to the boys, three young girls in parochial school uniform: lively eyes imprisoned in masks that promise obeisance, their movements a few steps beyond animation into rebound hyperactivity.

A fattish black boy in a schoolyard pushes all the smaller boys he can reach off their feet. Some of them cry, but he doesn't pay attention. In a corner, another little black boy sits pensive, alone. He sucks the thumb of one hand while he twirls his hair with the other.

A coffee shop full of early adolescent Eskimos: the girls all wear pink curlers in their hair, the boys in white leather jackets are droop-lidded on some kind of dope. They are town dwellers. In an isolated village much farther north, the children have happy, active faces. There the boys wrestle with their dogs and it is difficult to tell who enjoys the play more. The games are contests among hunters-to-be, throwing elongated sticks for distance, using their sling shots to fell birds.

Lassitudinous children in Haiti, the flies playing around their infected eyes. They will soon be frozen into the begging posture with outstretched hands. For the hope of a penny, they will sit in the sun for hours, waiting for the emergence of the tourist in the library. Their faces are pinched, hopeless.

Two small sisters in a clinic: their dresses freshly ironed. They are little dolls whose function is to be polite and stay freshly pressed.

A young Masai, earrings dangling from the hollowed extension of his ear lobes, three or four years away from circumcision and warrior status. He walks with grace, spear in hand, tending his herd. His bearing bespeaks the competence to deal with a meddling lion. He talks softly, smiles easily and moves like the others of his tribe, with dignity. Of all the gadgets we display, the only one that interests him are the binoculars, which enable him to make out details on distant hills that his sharp eyes cannot reach. In the songs at night his people always leave space for the full, deep expiration.

A bright ten-year-old sits serenely and with unassuming command as his mother, near to losing control of her voice, tells the psychiatrist how he has refused to eat anything but pretzels and crisp bacon for the past two weeks.

The too-goody little girl on my couch, whom I have painstakingly tortured for weeks and who has responded only with silent tears and forbearance, suddenly spins around and hisses, "Drop dead, you rat."

What conclusions can one draw about the nature of the species with such a variety of style, circumstance and performance? One fact is evident: whatever is the basic nature of the human animal, the societal pressures are a large force in determining what it becomes. And though many excoriate the industrialized societies for having plundered the world and the inhabitants thereof, a simple inspection of a primitive, superstitious, warring, sex-negating New Guinea society makes it clear that we are not the only villains. Once people dreamed that retreating into the simple world of the "noble savage" would restore us, pristine, into the bosom of nature -- an idea now thoroughly discredited. An antithetical view has been espoused by some in the Judeo-Christian tradition. Rather than seek for a state of natural grace by relaxing the structures of civilization, they proclaim that man is born in sin and must, from the moment of his birth, be hewn and shaped into a vessel more consistent with God's image.

Freud, armed with the data gleaned in his work, viewed the problem of man's nature and the relationship of the individual to his society as a two-edged sword. On the one hand, as Freud penetrated the social veneer, he engaged the unconscious with its polymorphous perverse sexuality and its destructive, homicidal impulses. This bestial, brutal, inner man had to be contained if the society were to function productively and peaceably. On the other hand, the conflict between the repressing forces and the repressed was the source of man's neurosis. One was faced with the choice between a ceaseless internal civil war or a brutish humanity. The choice was clear: one opted for the civilized society and bore the consequences.

But what of that vicious, uncivilized unconscious; is it not a fact? Yes, but it's a fact whose significance can be misinterpreted unless it is examined in the context of the conditions in which it exists.

To perform this examination, we can start in two places: with the infant as he grows and develops or with the patient as he proceeds in therapy.

When we examine the infant, we move in the direction of development and accretion. When we engage in the therapeutic procedure, we unpeel layers and in some sense move backward in time.

The first procedure: the newborn lies before us. She does not appear particularly vicious, kind, selfish, generous, secretive, nosey, or much else that pertains to morally desirable or undesirable traits. We can say that she is either an active or a quiet child, that she cries a lot or little, that she responds acutely or diffidently, that she sleeps most of the day or in short naps. At this point we can make no judgments on her behavior. She simply is an alive animal. She is not, however, a blank tablet. When we put her to a reactive breast, she snuggles in, breathes fully and is at ease. If we remove her from the breast while she is busily engaged in feeding, her face contorts, she yowls, her legs kick, her arms move about and her fingers contract. She is clearly displeased and she expresses her displeasure. She reacts to what suits her and what does not suit her. She has her own direction, her unique spirit. When she is frustrated, she is angry; but at this point we would be no more inclined to call her vicious or bestial than we would the puppy who tooths on our finger.

She grows -- one year, two years. She crawls underfoot, grabs for whatever she can reach, asserts herself in every possible circumstance. She has arrived at an age at which she is a conscious entity, and she affirms her individuality by constant opposition to direction from outside. She is aggressive, celebrating the year of "no." To keep her from interfering with her parents' routines, they consigned her to a playpen; and when, by some unimagined effort, she manages to escape, they whack her and place her back in quarters. She screams and throws tantrums, but her efforts only bring stiffened adult resistance and more antipathy. At length, she bends and learns to play quietly in her playpen. But now she is more restless at bedtime, talks of monsters who appear at the dark of night, demands that her room be lit for sleeping. Years later, when an investigating psychologist asks her to draw a person, she delineates a stick figure with stumps of arms and legs, indicating that she is no longer overtly aggressive, and stiletto fingers, indicating that her unconscious is now murderous. As time goes by, her overt fears may be quieted, her inner rage no longer projected in the monster image. It is now diffused in covert craftiness, distrust, tight-bellied withholding, stiff-necked obstinacy, masked facies and the superficial observance of compliance. She is complete.

Theory

Proceeding from the other direction, we examine our patients on the couch. Most of them are good citizens, "nice" people who make their way through life more injured than injuring -- on the conscious level. Occasionally one meets an exception, a political revolutionary, say, with a thinly veiled hatred and destructive bent for all mankind except those few colleagues he calls comrades. (This is not to imply that every revolutionary is hateful.) But he and the whiney girl with a vinegar face and bitter humor and several other "hostile" types are not so different from the "nice" patients. They all respond with anxiety when therapy releases the intense rage in their armored muscles. All patients on the couch, with the exception of some psychotics and psychopaths, defend themselves against their murderous rage.

The difference in the "nice" and "hostile" patients, then, is largely one of surface. The therapist irritates the surface differently to pierce the armor; for example, one might attack the superficial facade of the "nice" people from the psychological side, imitating their nice voice or their nice smile until they are provoked to anger, or one might attack the muscular armoring painfully, to the point where it brings out their angry resistance. With the overtly hostile patients, the path to the deep anger might be even longer. One might discover that the surface irritability is a defense against the pain or rejection by a cold father. Further on, we might come to the patient's longing to be loved by that father, then fear of him, and then, beneath all this, the vicious, destructive hatred toward him.

The layer of savage hate is usually there. Consistent work on the superficial armoring confirms the psychoanalytic finding that there is a beast in man, or, in fairness to our animal cousins, there is "evil" man in civilized man. However, having uncovered the brute, that is neither the end of therapy nor the end of the story.

As the patient repeats the expression of deep rage, as he becomes able to express it more fully and with less anxiety, his armoring softens and tends to disappear. Using facial armoring as an example, we would start with a patient whose face was a pleasant mask. In working past the defensive function of that mask, we would have discovered the savage face with hard lines, tight jaw and hateful eyes. But as therapy proceeds, the face softens -- particularly if lower segments have been loosened, the patient is in a position to tolerate his genital sensations and has a partner with whom he can express his sexual love. Later in therapy, as an exercise, he is free to express his rage, but the abiding affect is no longer there. His anger is mobile; it is expressed and gone. Now he is the vehicle of angry emotion when it is appropriate; he is no longer an angry person. His face is soft, mobile. It expresses what he feels at any particular moment -- anger, sadness, fear, joy, brightness. It is not a mask of anything.

If we have succeeded with our patient, you will search hard to find the beast in his unconscious. Conflagrations and explosions will no longer be his nightly store of dreams. Though we never completely rid ourselves or our patients of armoring, we at least approximate the state of simple aliveness of young children and puppies who have received considerate treatment. The unarmored individual may not be "nice," but he is decent.

This brief excursion, forward and backward, sketches in the layers of armoring that characterize most of us. The actual stratification of armoring is far more complicated than we have described. Each aspect may serve a simultaneous expressive and defensive function. One meets an affective expression at one level associated with one set of relationships, then confronts it again at a deeper level with another set of associative references. If one were to draw the laminations of armoring, the picture would resemble the confused geological strata following volcanic eruption. Nonetheless, three functionally distinct layers can always be distinguished.

The most superficial level of armoring is that of the social facade. This level varies widely in its manifestations. It includes demeanors of pleasantness, pertness, sweetness, curtness, churlishness, feigned stupidity and dismay, postures of thoughtfulness, aloofness, *Weltschmerz* -- and a thousand others. We are not speaking here of genuine, natural sweetness or innate thoughtfulness or sincere expression of pain but of the affected, counterfeit display of these attitudes.

This superficial layer of character has wandered farthest from its biological core and bounds the area where the individual merges with the social scene. Yet even here the biological signals are used -- the quiet voice that renounces aggression, the slack jaw that promises not to bite, or the squared jaw set on square shoulders to emphasize toughness.

The superficial layer is the one designed to represent us in the world. The amazing fact is not that the deceit works successfully so often on other armored personages (not with very young children or unneurotic animals), but it is the way we come to view ourselves for much of the time. Except for occasional lonely lapses into honest self-assessment, the vibrato-voiced cleric, the purse-lipped physician, the vocal philanthropist, the high-school sweetheart are themselves convinced by the act.

But we do not have the same feelings about the part of our character represented in the next layer, the secondary layer. Here reside those traits and impulses represented in the psychoanalytic unconscious. The adjectives we use to describe these characteristics -- bestial, savage, animal, brutish -- put distance between us and them; they are not of me, they are of another kind of creature. In reality they are a deeper, truer part of us than the qualities that defend us against them, the false qualities of the superficial character layer. All patients will fight mightily to keep the secondary layer from being unmasked. Even those who come to therapy proclaiming, "I am a bitch," will fight furiously to keep from making affective contact with the secondary layer. Their self-negating proclamations are a contactless veil to defend themselves against touching their devil.

There is a dilemma concerning the origin of the evil in men. We speak of original sin, yet we are aware of the "innocence of babes." Experience teaches us that "we are all sinners," yet we were "born in God's image." What transpired in the interlude between innocence and sin? Is there, as the story says, a villainous act in this piece -- the voice of the serpent (sexuality), eating of the fruit of the tree of knowledge (self-perception)?

To answer these questions, we must return to observations of the growing infant and pay particular attention to points of behavioral change.

We have said that the very young child is amoral, the vessel of drives, impulses and reactions. Some of the drives are present from birth (for example, sucking), and some increase to a critical point with the passage of time (for example, genital primacy). Probably a genetic endowment determines the energy level and broad outlines of personality structure (feisty, serene, etc.) with which the newborn enters the world, though the intra-uterine environment may play a larger role in this than we now know. The growing infant clearly displays preferences and is aggressive in expressing them and his displeasure when they are ignored. Unless the infant is consistently denied, the aggression increases with time.

Aggression is not an emotion, per se. It is a vehicle, a muscular readiness to satisfy emotional needs. In the newborn, the aggression is displayed by voice, facial expression and uncoordinated movement of extremities and trunk. Later the facial expression becomes more focused; and as the limbs become more finely tuned in purposive motion, they assume a larger burden of aggressive expression. Those unfamiliar with infant behavior need only watch the young child learning to take his first steps. He steps out, falls, rises and steps, falls, picks himself up, steps and falls again, and repeats this process thirty times past the time that an adult would have become discouraged and remained sitting.

The intact aggressiveness marks the child's style and spirit. So long as the aggression remains whole, the child remains vital and true. Let me hasten to add that the principle of not interfering with the child's natural aggression has nothing to do with standing by while the child hacks the furniture. The child destroys the furniture either innocently, in which case he must be instructed that it is not his right to destroy other's property, or out of meanness, which is a sign that his natural aggression has already been crippled. Chopping the furniture does nothing to express the child's natural needs.

When he asks questions about the world which is unknown to him, the consistent and straightforward answers to those questions sustain his aggressive need to know. The complete and timely satisfaction of his sucking needs maintains the aggression orally. Returning his deep gaze with one's open, feeling look preserves his aggressive need to make contact. Giving him rein to move about as freely as he is capable, to feel and find and manipulate (taking care to have removed all potentially harmful objects from his reach) supports his aggressive need to explore his world. Permitting him to express his displeasure by crying, and attempting to correct the situations that displease him, so long as they do not interfere with the rights of others, lets him know that he has an aggressive, meaningful voice in his affairs. Sustaining him in his active pleasure in his genitals and respecting the privacy of his activity in his love relationships when he grows to that age keep his love and desire clean and lively. One reacts to him when he is aggressively social, insofar as time permits, and does not interfere when he is engaged in solitary enterprise. The maintenance of a child's aggression is anything but passive laissez faire; it requires parental love, energy and sacrifice.

When the child's aggression is maintained in all spheres, there is no sudden behavioral shift. Innocence is replaced not by superficial "niceness" and secret plotting, not by outward balkiness or meanness or silence, but by awareness.

Other parental attitudes toward the child's natural display lead to a different place. The parental inhibition of the child's aggression induces armoring. Not to permit the child to cry or scream or voice opposition creates armoring in the throat or oral segment. To limit the child's freedom of movement leads to armoring of the shoulders and extremities. To fail to reciprocate with gaze induces armoring in the eye segment. To ignore the child's questions or to give silly or lying answers establishes armoring in the brain (eye segment). By failing to satisfy the oral needs, we create an armored mouth; and by failing to permit the development of self-regulated toilet patterns, we armor the rectum and anus. The inability to tolerate the child's natural sexuality destroys the innate sexual aggression and leaves an armored pelvis in its place.

At the point at which armoring is established, we note a radical alteration in behavior. The baby denied the returned gaze of recognition, acceptance and warmth gradually looks less intently. The eyes lose intensity and sparkle, interest decreases, the general energetic level is throttled. The baby may become cranky or irritable. He is different from the born child. The child deprived of free exploration gradually learns to live quietly in the crib or playpen, but there are new outbursts of tantrums or breath-holding, and the eyelids contract over so slightly into what will become the plotter's look. The child denied the pleasure of sweet-touching his genitals will suddenly move his hands above covers when his mother appears. He will sneak the feel henceforth and he will sneak feels with his girls. With armoring, innocence is gone and in its place, the human we all know -- the man Reich called homo normalis.

Homo normalis is divided -- divided into his conscious being and his typical Freudian unconscious. From an orgonomic perspective, he is divided into superficial, secondary and core levels of character functioning.

What is the mechanism of the abrupt swing from simple, straightforward unarmored functioning to the perverse functioning of the armored individual? It can be illustrated graphically by means of the following diagrams. The unarmored individual functions as in Fig.A

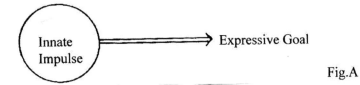

Fig.A

The armored individual can no longer function in a straight line because the goal is not tolerated in his environment, and he has armored against expressing it. The path that he is forced to follow

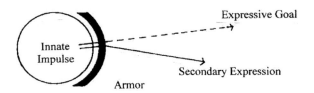

Fig. B

When his free, aggressive motoric explorations meet the armoring block, they are refracted from the original direction and become hateful aggressive displays (or the unconscious desire to hurt): The impulse to love tenderly and passionately is bent away from its goal by armoring and becomes sadistic sex, athletic sex, pornographic sex. The secondary layer contains the characterologic product of armored functioning. It is not innate. It is a "normal" artifact in a sick society.

Without armoring, the mind would have its unconscious aspect, which would operate on the principle of primary process (the place of origin for innate impulses), as it does now. But it would not be filled with the rage, longing, unfulfilled needs and sexual sickness, as it is with us. It would still be the vehicle of solving problems and would connect us with our primitive, creative core.

The ultimate, elemental inside of our character is the core layer. It is our source of feeling and action. When one is functioning from the core, one is emotionally vibrant, inventive, straightforward and considerate in relationships, in touch with oneself and the world. Core contact (at least part-time) is the source of artistic productions. It was preserved in inordinate measure in the child Mozart, in Mendelsshon, Macauley and Gauss. The point of orgonomic therapy and the disarmoring process is to get closer to core functioning.

The essential difference between functioning from the core layer and functioning from the secondary and superficial layers is that in the former the functioning is unitary and in the latter, divided. In the core layer, the meaning and the goal are true to the impulse of the source and are what the individual says they are. In the other, there is a split between impulse and effect, and dissimulation may be consciously or unconsciously involved. We are in the realism of the "kindnesses" that destroy, or "I do this for your good," of the caress that bruises, of rationalizations for deeds not performed.

This schism in character is the *fons et origo* of the artificial dualities with which our minds and behavior are seized. We set up a line of division between mind and body. We distinguish between what is spiritual and what is animal in us; we set-up an opposition between religion and sexuality. We array nature on one side of a fence and culture or civilization on the other. Work, devoid of invention and satisfaction, becomes the antithesis of pleasure.

Because of the split in ourselves, when we contemplate our world, we behold it from two opposed aspects. The mechanistic side declares that the cosmos, the world, our life -- all function according to the principles of mechanical law. We and our planet are machines. Discover the laws and tighten the bolts, and we shall proceed hummingly. No mysteries -- the answer will surely be discovered in the future. No emotional outbursts -- there's no need to get excited. Only efficiency! The complete mechanist solidifies his view by successfully eradicating any significant contact with his core. Emotions are successfully "handled" and he is free to follow his personal blueprint and to project his self-image upon the world.

On the other hand, the mystic eschews the solid things of this world and is preoccupied with the subtleties and mysteries of the forces behind the known phenomena. To him only the ethereal is significant; solidity is a distraction. The mysteries are never approached as problems to be solved, but only grazed from a wide tangent, taking care to keep them unknown. One must never get closer than metaphor.

There is a purpose in this mystique. Examination of patients with this bent reveals that, unlike the mechanists, they do maintain a limited contact with their inner emotional core. However, they cannot abide full and direct perception of their sexual feelings. To endure the contact, they must change its direction, project it into the heavens outside or to the "third eye" in the middle of their forehead -- as far from the genitals as possible. With the true source disguised, they are free to thrill -- safely.

We have described the poles of mechanistic and mystical behavior. The pure cultures of behavior are rare as pure races. The mechanist reserves Sunday for "things of the spirit" and the mystic enjoys his Mercedes. Each assumes that by dealing with matters both physical and spiritual, he is tapping the full range of existence. In truth, these are but two aspects of the distortion which armoring imposes.

Mechanism has its proper place in the world. It is the precise modality for dealing with what pertains to mechanistic physics. One would hesitate to enplane on a jet aircraft constructed on other principles. Regarding our bodies, mechanistic law relates to such matters as hydrostatic pressure in closed cylindrical systems (blood pressure), the functions of valves (some types of cardiac disorder) and gaseous exchange along membranes (respiration). Mechanical functions must be adequately maintained, but mechanistic law has no relevance to the quality of life. The quality of life is the province of orgone energy, which obeys its own laws.

Mystical thought recognizes the inadequacy of the mechanistic explanation of life and poses an alternative which is equally inadequate, for lack of substance. Mechanism and mysticism are like two argumentative old men, each of whom clearly sees the emptiness of his opponent's argument but fails to recognize the hollowness of his own.

The truth in the mystical view is that there is an extra-mechanical force at work in the universe. It has nothing to do with good and evil, "sin" and "grace," as the mystics would have it. The mystic's concept of sin is rooted in sexual guilt, but the natural world does not hang from this peg. In a consonant world one would redefine "sin" and "grace" (since these words have such popular appeal, we would retain them for friendship's sake). Sin is that which defies the order of nature. Consequently, to predicate sexual union on the issuance of a certificate by the marriage bureau rather than on the natural affection of lovers is a sin; to keep a baby from screaming when it is outraged is a sin; to stay married when all warmth has departed from the relationship is a sin; to fail to exercise one's mind or one's body sufficiently is a sin. In nature it is not necessary to wait for the afterlife for the punishment for sin; the penalty is almost immediate -- in the loss of fullness of life and diminished satisfaction in one's days. We can carry the mystical and real definition of sin one step further and speak of original sin. As the mystics speak of it, original sin is the cloud we are all born under in remembrance of the sexual transgressions of our ultimate ancestors, Adam and Eve. In reality, original sin has no moral overtones. It is the armoring which is imposed on us early in life by our armored parents -- all of us, we and they, innocent victims.

We would define "grace" as harmony with nature. To be totally alive with one's senses, fully perceptive, emotionally unrestricted, to have a mind free to explore and make new connections and a strong, agile body is to live in a state of grace.

The mystics would shrink from this definition. "There is only talk of self," they would say. "What of charity, sacrifice, kindness?" The answer is that in an armored world precepts must be established to dissuade us from the "evil" of the secondary layer. Where there is no secondary layer, there is no virtue (with moral overtones), but neither is there selfishness. Recent evidence from ethology supports the view that we do not eat to live, we live to eat. In some far day we may have learned not that we must live in harmony to survive, but that we survive, living in harmony.

Chapter 7
Therapeutic Procedure

In its broadest context psychiatric orgone therapy can be defined as the influence of one energy system (that of the therapist) on another (that of the patient) in removing the blocks to the orgasm reflex. The definition is not violated by the fact that only a minority of patients arrive at the point at which the orgasm reflex occurs with some regularity. The real therapeutic situation for most patients is that in the search for the ultimate objective (orgasm reflex), impediments to freer functioning are overcome, symptoms disappear and the experience of life becomes richer and more serious.

As much as we long for it, therapy is not a miracle cure. When we come to therapy, some of us are like trees with badly bowed trunks. We cannot straighten the original bowing. But we can diminish the degree of curvature and enable them to grow straighter than they otherwise would. With the youngest and the most flexible, we can almost achieve straight growth. In our metaphor, the bowing of the trunk represents physical and characterologic armoring. If the armoring is firmly established, it cannot be completely removed in therapy. In optimal circumstances, the patient may function as if the armoring were not present. But in acute traumatic situations, the patient will tend to hold in the places where he had always held. If the therapy has been successful, the process need not continue beyond tendency into actuality. But the tendency indicates that a trace of the armoring still exists.

For the patient, therapy is hard work. It requires commitment and courage. It demands that he walk into the dark places that he avoided since infancy or early childhood. When poorly informed advisers tell patients that entering therapy is a matter of relying on a therapist and of abandoning "solving one's own problems," they could not be further from the truth. No human act is braver than facing one's anxiety.

Patients range in age from early infancy to old age. Psychiatric orgone therapy is unique among psychotherapies in that it treats infant patients directly. Where parental treatment of the child is the cause of the infant's armoring, this treatment must be discovered and corrected either by simple instruction, or by therapy directed to one or both parents. Armoring in the infant can often be corrected in one or two sessions; the armoring is not yet rigid and the infant usually has a goodly store of energy with which to work. Obviously the therapist does not apply the same degree of physical force to the infant's armoring that he employs in treating his adult patients. The measures are simpler because the infant has not yet built defenses against defenses, as adult patients have. The armoring is usually obvious and easily eliminated. Whether the armoring recurs depends on the persistence of the environmental factors that originally created it.

A mother brings her four-month-old daughter to therapy because she has been whiny and irritable for several weeks and her feeding has become fitful. The mother, who had been in therapy, functioned well through pregnancy and delivery and had enjoyed the first months of motherhood before the onset of the recent symptoms. The child's state distresses the mother not only because of her obvious discomfort, but also because the mother's fantasy of a flawless motherhood and an ideally "healthy" child has been punctured.

For several weeks before the onset of the child's symptoms the mother had experienced marginal but increasing frustration over her inability to spend the amount of time she desired with her baby and still perform her housewifely duties with the same efficiency as before. Her husband had not offered to assist her in caring for the child because he assumed that this was her responsibility entirely. She had not broached the matter with him because she anticipated that with increased experience she would be able to handle things adequately. Her throat, which had been a significant area of armoring during her therapy, is again armored. Clearly she is repressing frustration and anger in her effort to fit the myth of perfect and sublime motherhood. With its sensitive perception, the child has picked up on the mother's repression to the point where symptoms have erupted.

As I examine the infant, I can see that her chest is not moving freely, her neck is slight rigid and the sounds that she makes are being squeezed through an armored throat. Otherwise there is no significant armoring. The eyes are open, lively and trusting, the abdomen is soft, the pelvis freely movable.

I instruct the mother to hold the infant and scream with almighty rage. When she does, the infant opens her eyes wide and gazes at the mother with a look of startled disbelief. Then she, too, begins to cry and scream. The session is terminated at the point at which the infant's scream expresses the full frustration of her condition.

In the following week the mother reports that the whining and irritability never recurred after the therapy session. The infant is again feeding with her usual gusto. The mother has returned home and instituted a new familial *modus vivendi* in which the husband participates in household and child-caring tasks. The emotional air in the house is brighter. The state of motherhood in that household is now less "perfect" but more real.

The patient is a bright, gentle four-year-old with armoring of the ocular segment that is going to require painful pressure to eradicate. I approach her with some trepidation. This is our first meeting and I would prefer not to hurt her; but as I observe her flattened expression, I put that preference aside. I proceed to prod deeply in the forehead and temple area and elicit cries, yells and ultimately the straight-forward facial expression of fury directed at me. She spends her wrath punching at me and is finally satisfied. Now her eyes are sparkling and her face is alive. On her way out from the treatment room through my office, she stops in her tracks, makes a detour behind my desk and gives me a broad, frank kiss.

The frustrating factor in the treatment of children is the reappearance of armoring once it has been cleared, due to environmental conditions beyond the child's control. If the conditions that created the armoring continue to prevail, the armoring will reemerge despite treatment. Consequently, parental guidance or treatment is often the crucial fact in the child's treatment. Once the child has grown to adolescence the significance of parental influence declines, but before that time the fact of the child's dependence is critical.

The treatment of adolescents is generally undertaken only in the face of severe problems. Puberty is such a time of change and upheaval that one interferes only to keep the patient afloat and off the shoals. One doesn't embark on long therapeutic journeys in such rough seas and shifting winds. The surest course is to intervene only when necessary, removing the most obvious armoring, then to take one's hands off and give the person a chance to find his own way.

The treatment of aged patients is usually assumed for purposes of symptomatic relief. Generally armoring becomes "institutionalized" with age, the person has accustomed himself to an equilibrium in which the armoring is a significant factor, and one intervenes only when the equilibrium becomes disestablished, precipitating symptoms.

A seventy-eight-year-old woman has made an uneventful recovery from major surgery, but she has become acutely anxious about falling. Her anxiety is so severe that she is afraid to venture onto her feet. She is lying with fixed eyes, tight upraised shoulders, stiff and barely moving chest. Her pupils are wide, extremities cold.

I gently encourage her to freer breathing. Once the chest is mobilized, we work on eye movement, which she tries fearfully at first, then with increased confidence. When the eyes move relatively freely, we speak of her fear of dying -- a fear that struck her with full force after the surgical emergency had been met. She felt in such danger of dying that only by assuming a state of almost complete immobility, the paralysis defense of the cornered animal, could she hope to escape the attention of the angel of death.

Now, with her eyes and chest mobile, I gently encourage movements of the shoulders and arms in the sitting position. She is more comfortable now and beginning to be at ease in her surroundings.

At the next session her anxiety is considerably decreased. Her daughter reports that during the week she has occasionally ventured from the room unassisted. The eyes, chest and shoulders are mobilized again, and I instruct her to kick in the supine position (lying on her back), with the aim of getting energy into her legs, giving her more assurance of their solidity. She is more lively and cooperative at this second meeting. Her daughter calls on the following week to report that her mother is now moving about freely. No vestige of the falling anxiety remains.

In treating patients, one generally proceeds from the head downward to the pelvis. There are two reasons for this procedure: First, armoring in a higher segment binds energy that is necessary for the dissolution of the armoring in the lower segment. And second, the deepest and most frightening anxiety (sexual anxiety) resides in the pelvic segment and one does not begin to deal with this anxiety until the individual has gained energy and emotional strength from having dealt with the anxieties of the higher segments.

The first task of treatment is to determine the location and intensity of the armoring, then to discover how it fits in the pattern of defenses of the patient. Therapy is a detective operation. One does not merely discover a layer of armoring, treat it, discern the next holding place and loosen it. Unless therapist and patient slowly and painstakingly relate the function of one defensive operation to the next -

- that is, discover the architecture of the defensive system -- they have not solved the problem of the character structure, and the loose ends will produce pathology of one sort or another.

Providing dramatic episodes in therapy is relatively simple; but, except for the transitory effect of the positive transference which the drama provides, it achieves little of lasting value. In some cases, the flashy effect has itself become an agent of the defensive system, standing in the way of significant movement or discovery. Thus, inexperienced, too-adventurous therapists have reported on cases in which the orgasm reflex was elicited on the first or second therapeutic session, and the patient was so frightened that the reflex did not reappear for years -- or ever. One does not foreswear all dramatic episodes in therapy. There is a natural drama in every life, and from time to time it surfaces in therapy, unprodded and unprovoked. The excitement of new discoveries and recovered memories stimulates further therapeutic progress, but the essential movement of therapy owes more to the thoughtful step-by-step advance due to hard work than to the occasional leaps.

The therapist locates the armoring by observing the patient at his ordinary activity, then in the performance of specific emotional tasks. For example, as the patient talks to you, you note that he averts his gaze, or that his eyes are blank or too animated. You watch him play with his fingers. His trunk is ramrod stiff on the chair, or he slouches. He smiles whenever he speaks of things that provoke anxiety, or his eyes become dulled momentarily. His handshake is reactively aggressive, or flabby, or you feel that he really senses and values the contact.

These impressions and many more add up to an initial evaluation of the individual's status. The experienced therapist knows that the armoring that he uncovers early in therapy does not define the entire gamut of armoring in the patient. Areas that appear free of armoring on superficial inspection will become regions of blockage as the therapy progresses. But these areas of armoring will be dealt with in their time.

In general, each segment of armoring may contain traces of superficial and secondary armoring; once the armoring is dissipated, the core function of the segment is revealed. For example, one would work through the meaning of sad, pleading eyes in the superficial layer, arrive at the frustration and anger that occasioned the sadness and pleading, and only after the secondary layer of anger is fully expressed would the eyes be capable of expressing the warmth and trust which was their elemental property. The foregoing model is a gross simplification of the process as it unwinds in the actual therapeutic experience. In some segments the secondary is already clearly revealed -- for example, in angry jaws or clenched fists -- and it is not necessary to work through the superficial layer. The meaning of the superficial layer in these instances is simple inhibition.

In each armored segment, the angry uses of the segment's affect generally come out before the tender emotions. There are two reasons for this: First, that is the way the emotions are layered. And second, so long as any vestige of secondary layer emotion is present, one cannot reach the deepest tenderness and openness. The lingering traces of anger lurk in the shadow, warning against complete exposure. The exception to this rule is when a patient has been sorely injured and abused in his life and is closed off to all relationships. The only hope of any progress in therapy lies in the establishment of sufficient warmth and trust between patient and therapist to enable him to open up to another person.

Every patient is unique. No case is easy (except in some instances where the goal is merely symptomatic relief). The patient is always wiser in the employment of his defenses than the therapist is in discovering them.

Whether the therapist addresses himself initially to a discussion of character traits he has observed or begins with work on the physical armoring is a matter of the propriety in the individual case. Some patients are so delicate that one does not put them on the couch for months, not until they are shored-up sufficiently so that the physical work is not threatening. Other patients in whom the physical armoring is so obvious and so symptomatically troublesome are treated immediately from the physical side. Whether the therapist approaches the patient first from one side or the other makes no difference; in either event he is working on the character structure. Therapy is not a matter of doing a little physical work, then doing a little talking, as some who are ignorant of the process assume. It is always a matter of working on the character structure wherever it can most easily be grasped. Of the psychoanalytic techniques, the only one that is employed with any frequency is dream interpretation, and then not in the meticulous weeks-long search for the associations of each element as in the psychoanalytic manner, but in a more general, intuitive way to discern signposts in the unconscious.

The idiosyncratic patterns of defense are exemplified by the following three patients, each of whom is hiding sadness.

The first is a witty, vivacious student in her early twenties who is never silent. She is bursting with energy, attractive, constantly on the move. On the couch in her first session I forbid her to talk. I ask her to breathe easily but freely. She follows instructions, and after several breaths she raises her finger, indicating that she has something to say. I place her upraised finger down by her side and say that she should go on breathing. After a dozen more breaths the finger rises again, and her eyes and a humming sound indicate that she has something really important to communicate. I replace her finger by her side and repeat the instructions. One final attempt to talk is parried, and by this time she realizes that the ploy will not work. She proceeds more seriously with the breathing now, and in a short time she is crying in sobs that overwhelm her. The vivacity has been exposed as the distraction from her sadness. She cried subsequently in each therapeutic hour for weeks.

The second patient, also in her twenties, is tough and cynical. She works in advertising, which helps to reinforce her classification of her species -- "those who take and those who are taken." She is not one of the taken.

In therapy she is constantly demanding and critical: I am not sufficiently inventive. I am thinking of other things while I am treating her. We always do the same thing; not enough is happening. To my answer that everything that she does is mechanical she replies that that's the only way she can do what I ask. After weeks of her harangue, I arrive one day at the break point and lash out at her, concluding with an invitation to leave therapy. Her demeanor changes immediately and she cries deeply, murmuring, "I'm sorry, I'm sorry." Now she is no longer a tough, slick woman, but a whimpering, sad little girl. Her offensive defense has been cracked, exposing the misery beneath.

The third patient, in his late twenties, is the most amusing patient I have known. His stories are so funny that I must discipline myself to cut him off so that we can get work done. Even on the couch he often interrupts with a humorous insight that sets us both laughing. He is at the beginning of a career as a professional comic and has achieved some acclaim. In fairness to him, I recognize that we cannot continue in this manner. At great personal loss, I inform him that henceforth there must be no humorous talk between us. He is an essentially serious man and he accepts the prohibition soberly. Now his demeanor in therapy is changed. He is uncomfortable, ill at ease. He makes a few attempts at jests, but stops himself. With work on his throat and chest, we soon arrive at a deeper level of crying than we had achieved before. The sadness deepens and continues with time. He says that he has to work harder at being funny now because he usually feels sad. The jocular subterfuge no longer works. He ultimately gave up comedy for another profession.

The combination of being deprived of the defenses of the superficial layer and of increasing the energy level by full breathing is usually sufficient to propel submerged, repressed feelings toward the surface. The beginning therapist, armed with a bag of clever tricks, is sometimes eager to demonstrate his prowess by "jumping in and making things happen." If he succumbs to the temptation, he only muddies the waters. In most cases the simple expedient of permitting the patient to do nothing but breathe more fully starts him in the direction of unraveling. The two qualities that the understanding American obstetrician, Dr. Joseph deLee, described as desirable in the obstetrician apply to the medical orgonomist in the onset of treatment. "He should have," Dr. deLee said, "a set of fat buttocks; and he should know how to sit on them." The therapist's willingness to stand aside after applying slight pressure to the repressed side of the patient's character structure permits the emergence of emotions in an orderly, comprehensible fashion, so that the architecture of the character can ultimately be discerned. In the final analysis, one must depend on the patient for his own progress, and here, in the beginning, is a good place to start.

Having made a foray into the character depths on the initial visit, the therapist anticipates seeing some change on the next one. The patient returns, and there may be some observable difference in his attitude. But also there may not be. He may find that although at the last visit the patient was a body of fuming emotion, he is now his original, stock-still, contained, dead self. There is not a scratch, not a faint scar of the wound exposed in the previous session. He is "restored." Moreover, when he is put on the couch and the same pressures are applied, nothing happens. He is not merely reconstituted, he is reinforced! Character, in an attempt to maintain the so-long-held equilibrium, has increased the defensive array against change. One may work for the next five visits to attain the degree of opening of the first session. The battle lines are drawn.

Why, since the patient's life is so troubled that he has sought professional help, and since it is obviously in his interest to cooperate fully, does he invariably throw up such formidable resistance to progress?

A patient on whose cervical armoring we are concentrating gives one answer. Her armoring is that of stubbornness, and she and I have had revelations of the wild rage beneath the stubborn defense. We both know, too, the difficulties that her stubbornness has gotten her into in her life. At one point I say in exasperation, "Why don't you stop being so dammed stubborn?" And she yells in reply, "Because to me that's me. It's the only me I know; and I'm afraid that if I weren't stubborn, I'd be nothing!"

When the alternatives are maintaining the character defense or facing a feared ego disintegration, it is no wonder that patients apply Herculean efforts in resisting.

Other, more subtle examples of resistance:

A patient has just been through a screaming tantrum that was partly mechanical, but contained some elements of affect. Afterwards I ask, "What did you feel?" He replies with a clear note of triumph, "Nothing." I challenge the note of victory in his voice and point out that if he really felt nothing, he should be disappointed rather than triumphant. Following this path, we discover that it is more important for him to defeat me than to open up his depth. From here we get to the anger that is blanketed by his affectlessness.

An early middle-aged man is breathing down through the diaphragmatic segment without resistance. "This sure is a great feeling," he says as he continues. In a short time he announces, "I want to rage now, O.K.?" "No, just keep on as you are." He continues for several minutes more, then informs me that "there's some rage that has to come out." I tell him to "cool it." After several more minutes he says, "I'll tell you the truth, that feeling down there is driving me nuts."

A regular feature of therapy is the discovery of accented armoring of a lower segment once the armoring of a higher segment has been cleared. It is as if the enemy marches from head to pelvis; as the patient makes progress, the scattered defensive troops regroup and concentrate the more as therapy approaches the ultimate defensive position, the pelvic segment.

Sometimes areas which appeared to be unarmored in the initial evaluation become areas of strong resistance as the therapy progresses. For this reason, one cannot definitively specify the extent of armoring until the pelvic segment has been reached.

Not only does the armoring of lower segments increase as higher armoring is dissolved; but when one is at work on the armoring of the lower segment, the armoring in the higher segment often reappears, like the reemergence of a brush fire in an already dampened area. The rekindled brush fire must then once again be stamped out before the work can proceed. This process often is repeated many times.

A woman in her mid-thirties, bland, faceless, is asked to make a face. Her response to this request is usually anger. But as she advances toward more complete expression of anger, she invariably becomes nauseated. We do not yet proceed with work on the armored diaphragm by practicing gagging for fear that loosening down that far would expose her to energetic forces that she could not tolerate. After months, she learns to express her anger more fully without becoming nauseated. Now her expression is more lively; she is more active, and friends compliment her on how well she looks. It is now safe to proceed with work on the armored diaphragmatic segment. We work on gagging for the entire session. At our next meeting she appears her old self -- her face has lost its expression and she is once again drained of energy.

Working through the emotion in any armored segment inevitably leads to the release of overt anxiety and a subsequent contraction. Contraction follows expansion (release, freedom) as inevitably as night follows day. The inability of the armored human being to tolerate states of emotional expansion is a fact of which revolutionary leaders and political quacks who promise "the liberation of mankind" (Reich called them "freedom peddlers") are unaware. In the course of therapy, every patient is at some point freed -- and cannot stand it! Then he crawls back into whatever refuge he has constructed in the course of his life and gazes longingly outward. It is not by chance that most men live "lives of quiet desperation." We dream of freedom from our shackles; but when they are taken from us, we grab for them because they have become part of us.

A borderline psychotic law student, who is in danger of flunking out of school, is expressing rage by punching and yelling. His throat suddenly tightens and he reaches for it with both hands as if to attempt to loosen the tight ring. He coughs repeatedly, and soon he is sobbing. The deep sobs come freely and he cries through most of the hour. When he is finished he says, "I can't remember crying since I was a tiny kid. That felt so great." He turns pale and begins to tremble. The tremors spread throughout his body. He dresses and pulls a cover around him, but the shaking is unabated. He sits in the waiting room through the session with the next patient; and when I see him at the end of that hour, he is still trembling though the intensity has declined. At his next session he reports that he shook intermittently throughout the week and had periods in which he thought he would faint. He says in half-jest, "You're a bigger son of a bitch than my last psychiatrist. He didn't do anything; you do something, and I'm worse-off than I was before."

For the patient, therapy is a constant process of reaching in for repressed emotions, finding and expressing them, enduring the period of anxiety following release, becoming comfortable again, then repeating the process with the next deeper anxiety, and on, till he reaches the deepest anxiety. In the course of treatment, the patient feels better, then worse, then better, then worse. In general, each good period is a little higher than the previous one, and he tolerates low periods better. This general rule does not hold for the final anxiety, pelvic anxiety, which is the most terrifying of all. In the period that patients face their sexual anxiety, they may feel worse than they ever remember and develop symptoms they never had before.

In the therapeutic pursuit from the top to the bottom segment, the therapist devotes special attention to the eye segment. Unless the armoring in the eye segment has been dealt with thoroughly, the effect of work on any other armored segment is attenuated. If the patient's eyes are dull, then he is incompletely involved in proportion to the dulling of the eyes. If his eyes express deceit and this expression escapes the attention of the therapist, then he will be fooled by the semblance of emotional expression in lower segments. If the eyes show disdain, cunning, distance, that, too, will interfere with the work below. Their eyes are the chief place of escape for the patient. The patient who plays bridge in her mind during sexual intercourse is fleeing in her eyes. Everyone who fantasizes when he makes love is escaping from his mate with his eyes. Full, clear, eye contact is necessary for total involvement. Consequently, throughout therapy one returns again and again to the eyes to insure that they are not used as a sanctuary from complete participation.

The eye (brain) segment is also the seat of rationalization -- which of course, has a prime place in every good neurotic defense. The rational uses of the brain have brought us encyclopedias and moon walks; the defensive uses of thought sequester us from our feelings and are enemies to affective flow in therapy. Analysis stops action, and for this reason the company of many psychoanalysts is often deadly dull. The fault of analyzing while in action is common to patients who have been in psychoanalysis. It is an added burden to the therapy. In medical orgonomy we refer to this kind of interference as brain parasitism; energy is withdrawn from its place of action (in the muscles) into the brain, and the action ceases.

Processes of depersonalization and dissociation have their origin in the withdrawal of energy into the head. There is a lack of charge and a disruption of the current of excitation in the rest of the body. The withdrawal of energy creates the sensation of standing outside one's body or being an observer of the action in which one is involved.

An example of the absurd lengths to which brain activity can be carried in interfering with the emotive process is exemplified by a medical student patient who, at the precise point at which he was about to burst into sobs, suddenly became intellectual, preoccupied with the physiology of the tear glands as they relate to emotion, and how they connect with the vocal cry.

The work on the oral and cervical segments does not involve the same kinds of intense watchfulness as work on the eye armoring. The ordinary rule of first dealing with the negative emotions before attempting to elicit the warm emotional expressions of the segment applies. One cannot get at the patient's warmth until he has acknowledged, expressed and felt the hateful feelings. The biting, growling, yelling and crying must be exorcised before the lips can suck with appreciation, the face smile openly and warmly and the throat make deep, modulated sounds.

The chest segment is extraordinarily important in therapy. As the patient begins each session, the first order of business always is to breathe freely with the chest. By increasing the intake and distribution of orgone energy, free breathing increases the energy level throughout the body and exerts pressure on armoring, wherever it exists. The armoring may not even be noticeable until full breathing begins. For example, one may observe nothing unusual in the patient's eyes until his breathing becomes full. Then we watch the eyes become increasingly dulled as the patient turns-off to the intolerable sensations of the higher energy level.

While breathing, patients often experience a sensation of tingling in various body parts, often in the extremities. Those trained in the medical or biological sciences immediately ascribe these effects to hyperventilation and assume that they have explained the phenomenon. The truth is that the classical descriptions of the physiology of hyperventilation only describe the sensory phenomena; they do not begin to explain them, except in terms of nerve and muscle hyperirritability (see Appendix). The connection between the chemical changes and the hyperirritability is never established.

Against the purely chemical explanation, note the following facts observed in therapy: There is usually a line of demarcation where the tingling stops. The tingling never penetrates into a heavily armored area. Once the armoring is dissolved out of a segment, the tingling continues into that area. Some patients take five full breaths and they are tingling all over. Others breathe an hour and feel little or no tingling. At the beginning of therapy, some patients experience intense sensations that lead to carpopedal spasm (curling of fingers and toes) -- a classical sign of hyperventilation. Later in therapy, when they can tolerate higher levels of energy, they can breathe much longer and fuller, and these things do not occur. Tingling sensations (also described as a numbness, humming, ice water in the blood) are uncomfortable to patients in a contracted, low-energy state, but they are stimulating and pleasant to more alive bodies.

The sensation is not confined to the treatment room. Emotionally alive individuals experience it during states of high emotion (tingling with excitement or pleasure), or when they are thrilled as by music or a vivid sunrise.

The treatment of armoring in the diaphragmatic segment is often time-consuming because the patient must surrender to his energetic flow, an act which is difficult to learn. Work through the diaphragmatic, abdominal and pelvic segments is more often concerned with giving-in to oneself, than with moving outward.

As one approaches the pelvic armoring, a complete review of the patient's sexuality is often in order. The patient goes over sexual guilt, sexual experiences from childhood and sexual fantasies. Sometimes these matters have been discussed before. At any rate, pathologic sexuality, both psychological and somatic, is finally cleared when the patient has dealt with his pelvic armoring. The result is that he experiences intense pleasure anxiety.

Pleasure anxiety is the inability to tolerate pleasurable sensations in the body. It is difficult to understand except by those who have experienced it. We all assume that we want as much pleasure as we can have. Then why are we unable to tolerate it?

The deepest and fullest animal pleasure is the uninhibited flow of energy into and through the genitals. In a society in which the full, deep experience of genital pleasure in childhood is equated with sin, where little boys and girls who have been discovered loving sexually are regarded as villains, a giant inhibition is interposed between the genital apparatus and the total in-pouring of energy. A certain level of energy is tolerated, and this is experienced as sexual gratification. When the energetic flow is higher than the tolerated level, anxiety is precipitated and the entire body joins in "no." The inflection of the "no" is terrifying. Patients give the following accounts:

"The other day I felt that I was almost going to come and suddenly I was yelling, "No, no," and I don't even know where it came from. I wasn't thinking it consciously."

"I start feeling soft and warm, and then I get scared and actually think I'm going to die. And I have to stop."

"The whole day I was feeling sexy, and near the end of work I was really looking forward to going home and rushing into bed with S. Then these strong feelings started in my pelvis. They came in waves. One wave would start and it would go away, then another one, bigger than before, would come. I got so scared that I had a real bad anxiety attack, and by the time I got home I was a wreck."

"You know my trick of traveling around to various places in my head when I'm making love. Well, last week I followed your instructions and didn't do it. I just let myself concentrate on the feelings in my vagina, and it was marvelous. But just when I was about to have my climax, I let myself travel again. But this time I was in a place I didn't know and I was lost. I got so scared I pushed R. away and started to cry."

The time when the pelvic armoring is approached, which is called the end phase of therapy, is perilous. Patients frequently have acute anxiety attacks as well as falling anxiety and fear of dying. Men sometimes experience sexual impotence or penile anesthesia for the first time in their lives; women have frigidity and vaginal anesthesia.

During the end phase, in a desperate last-ditch effort not to submit, all the old armoring that had been cleared tends to reinsinuate itself -- and with vengeance. Somatic disorders sometimes develop in the armored segments. It is a time when, as one patient put it, "all the places have a chance to see what they remember." The therapist's attention is constantly distracted from work on the pelvic segment to long-gone armoring, now reinstituted. The body fights desperately against achieving full freedom, while the patient's energy gathers toward it.

Most patients do not achieve the regular appearance of the orgasm reflex in therapy. Of those who do reach this level, most must wait for a year or two after therapy before the reflex becomes a regular feature of the genital embrace. In this time they work through the lingering traces of anxiety in their daily lives and gain the courage to live deeply.

The majority of patients leave therapy or are discharged before they attain the level of full genitality. For the most part they came to therapy because their lives were distraught, or they were not performing efficiently, or they had distressing symptoms. Once they had broken through enough of their armoring so that these conditions changed, they often were not interested in more therapy; and for them the choice was correct. Some patients wish to continue further, but are discouraged by the therapist, who balances the current state of well-being against the strength of the remaining armor and the potential for anxiety with further therapy. Just as there are some patients whose armoring is so brittle that they are best not treated with orgone therapy, there are others for whom caution must overrule valor in deciding on continued therapy.

The treatment of each patient is a totally individual matter. One would try certain measures with one patient that would be unthinkable with another. Most patients are made to lie with legs extended, and the therapist corrects them when they cross their legs because this interferes with the energetic flow. But I do not even mention this to the schizophrenic boy whose legs are crossed in a tight knot because he is holding on to this side of sanity with all his might. For him, the abandonment of the pelvic defenses might tip the balance to psychosis. Nor do I discuss the defensive function of her fat with the obese girl who is barely coping with school, family and social pressures. We will discuss her fatty armoring at a later time when she is stronger. We deal with all armoring whether hypertonic (tense), hypotonic (flabby) or fat only when the patient has sufficient energy to handle it.

The energetic flow is something that the patient gathers in the course of time. Reich once compared the treatment of a patient to the progress of a locomotive through a mountainous area, where rocks had fallen onto the track. The therapist's function is to remove the rocks, not to push the locomotive. As the impedences are cleared, the momentum of the locomotive increases. With regard to the final block, the pelvic block, Reich cautioned, "You don't go down (to the pelvis); the down comes up to you."

The essence of good therapy is that it must be logical. There must be a consistent uncovering of the neurotic character patterns with a consequent enlargement of the patient's potential. In a misguided therapy, one might dig into a deep layer before the superficial debris had been removed and suffer a cave-in. Chaos would ensue. There are some therapies based very loosely on a Reichian model in which this situation pertains.

From time to time, a therapist may employ various devices as he works on the psychological or physical side of the patient's armoring. Reich experimented with the Medical DOR-Buster[14] to facilitate the breakdown of armoring; DOR (deadly orgone energy) is an energetic by-product of armoring. The DOR-buster is a modification of the orgone accumulator[15] (a device that increases the concentration of orgone energy above that which prevails in the atmosphere at large). The DOR-buster operates on the principle, discovered by Reich, that a metal tube, whose effects are exaggerated by an orgone energy accumulator which empties into fresh water, has the property of attracting concentrations of DOR into the water. No therapeutic claims are ever made to patients when theses devices are employed. Orgone accumulator devices are not prescribed in therapy, but some patients construct them and try them on their own. Their use is strictly in the investigative, experimental stage; and the scientific investigation of the physical orgone energy proceeds continually in laboratories here and

---

[14]Reich, Wilhelm, "The Medical Dor-Buster," *Core*, Volume VIII, No. 3-4, Dec., 1955.
[15]Reich, Wilhelm, *The Orgone Energy Accumulator, Its Scientific and Medical Use*, Orgone Institute Press, 1951.

abroad.   Hydrotherapy is occasionally recommended in states of agitation or listlessness.

Drugs are used in psychiatric orgone therapy, but not to the extent they are used in most psychotherapies.   The therapist may prescribe them when patients are in states of acute anxiety, but only if the level of anxiety is more than the patient can tolerate, and only with the understanding that this is a temporary expedient. The wholesale use of tranquilizers is decried in medical orgonomy. Anti-depressants are used in treatment of depression only when the therapy has not had enough time to take hold. Most depressions are treated with drugs only until the patient's structure can perform ist own healing.

The use of drugs in treatment of somatic disorders generally follows conventional medical practice.   Although orgonomic theory assumes that most somatic disorders, including cancer, are of biopathic origin -- that is, they are tissue disorders related to the armoring process -- many disorders, when they are full blown, are more amenable to treatment by conventional means than by work on the armoring, which was their source. This would vary with the potential for reversibility in the disorder. For example, a patient who came to therapy suffering from pylorospasm would continue to take his anti-spasmodic medication until the therapy had penetrated through the armoring of diaphragmatic and abdominal segments; then his pylorospasm should have been dissipated.

All patients are advised to exercise vigorously. Regular, hard exercise accomplishes two things. It aids in energy metabolism, providing a source of energetic discharge, so that the organism is then free to charge up to a higher degree. Secondly, it gradually increases muscle tone. Tonic musculature is capable of holding a higher charge than atonic musculature, so the patient will have a greater potential for work. From the psychological side, having a strong body makes one feel more capable and confident.   A confident patient will attack problems in therapy from which a less confident patient would flee.

Therapy is generally conducted once a week, sometimes twice weekly, and in times of crisis, more frequently as the situation demands. The duration of treatment varies widely. Symptomatic cures that appear dramatic are often achieved in one or two visits. On the other hand, there are patients who have been in therapy for five or seven years, and who continue because they are still making progress. Reich once declared that no patient should be treated for more than three years, assuming that after this time there were diminishing returns. But many therapists, acting in accord with their own experience, do not follow this rule. The logistics of the situation need to be considered. The demand for therapy greatly exceeds the number of qualified therapists. Does one proceed for another year with this patient, who will likely gain a half-inch, or does one take on a new patient, who will probably gain two inches?

Patients often take breaks from their therapy. They stay away for a period of months to years to enable their lives to catch up to the new capabilities of their character. When the therapist's annual vacation imposes a break, many patients report, "I didn't know that I could do this well without therapy." Others return and say, "I felt great while you were away; I think I'd like to stop now and see how it goes. If I need you, I'll call you." On most occasions, the therapist will give his blessing to the departure.

The integration of the therapeutic experience with the movement of life outside poses occasional problems. Reich once revealed that he sometimes would stop in the course of treating a patient and think, "This is an utterly weird activity in which to be involved; patients screaming and crying, punching the couch -- and out there deer are grazing. Sometimes," he said, "this seems like a strange kind of work to do, and sometimes it seems like the most important."

This is an experience shared, I am sure, by every therapist, and at some time in the course of therapy, by most patients. From one perspective, there is an ivory-tower quality to the therapeutic scene. In the world outside, simulation and superficiality are the ordinary modes; they are banned from the treatment room. The feigned smile may ease one's way through the social day, but on the treatment couch, it raises the therapist's hackles. More than one patient has remonstrated, "But it's not like that out there!" The objection is true, but unimportant. The therapeutic relationship does not seek to duplicate the social milieu, but to undo its damaging effects. The therapist knows that the patient must make his way in the world, but not at the peril of his soul.

Then there are the inevitable times when one is at work on the problems of armoring, and thoughts drift to the world outside. The mind wanders to the nightly danger in the streets, the benumbed mobs throughout the world, the fouled atmosphere, corrupt political systems and sick officials, and one wonders at a process that uncovers nature in the patient only to have it subjected to later assault at a hundred different levels. Occasionally the pressures of life are so acute that the patient must temporarily abandon the search into himself until the outside problem is settled.

For the most part, though, there is a confluence of therapy and life. Character is fate. Each increment to the patient's ability adds to his options. When his personal strength is enhanced, so is his ability to overcome obstacles. For example, if therapy makes one less tolerant of falseness and triviality and more discerning of the game-playing of suitors, thereby decreasing the number of potential mates, it also insures that one will not become caught in a flimsy relationship.

The goal of therapy is not for patients to be totally free of armoring at all times. A totally unarmored human in a heavily armored society is subjected to disdain, abuse and misunderstanding at every turn, and he suffers the ultimate fate of Dostoyevsky's Idiot. Armoring must be worn for selective occasions to prevent this fate. This type of armoring is flexible, worn like a coat rather than borne as an inflexible corset.

A young man suffers from a frightful obsessive disorder. Any reference to man's finite life causes him to become preoccupied with thoughts of death, sometimes for hours.

He is emotionally dry and appears to be dull, though he is not. In the two years of his therapy, there has been no sign of affect, nor any symptomatic change except for an increase in anxiety. In one session, the dam breaks; he not only sobs beyond control, but gives voice to his rage, crying, "I'll tell you one thing, if I ever kill myself I'm going to take a lot of people with me."

On the following visit he says, "You know the funniest thing happened after last week. I went home, I watched a TV program, and there were graves in it. Then I started talking to my parents about graves, but I didn't have any feeling about dwelling on it. I was just talking about death like a normal human being."

Symptoms are the ultimate manifestation of the pathological disorder; they are not the disorder itself. Beneath the symptoms are general reaction patterns, which are a step closer to the source. One patient never perspired before therapy; now she perspires profusely. Another patient had become so accustomed to "stronging it" (his words) to physical pain that his perception of pain had decreased to the point of bare recognition. Now things hurt again.

Dealing directly with energetic forces, psychiatric orgone therapy is powerful medicine. I remember feeling, after therapeutic sessions with Reich, that I had been propelled into another dimension, as if I perceived and functioned at a more intense level. I assume and hope that my patients have this same experience.

The therapy is employed in all disorders in which pulsation of the organism is disturbed. This encompasses a wide range of disturbance, including all functional emotional disorders (with the limitation that since most therapists are engaged in private practice the patient must be ambulatory and in sufficient contact to come to therapy) and all biopathies (physical disorders which arise from a disturbance of pulsation) which are not yet irreversible.

Chapter 8
Six Patients: Case Histories

In this section I shall describe segments of case histories, some single sessions and some longer stretches that illustrate principles of orgone therapy. I have purposely avoided detailing single-case histories from beginning to end because too often patients use them as models. Since everyone's therapy is unique, the stories are ultimately more misleading than helpful.

Case 1

A pale woman in her mid-thirties with a little girl voice, little girl body, dead eyes and stiff mouth (I omit reference to the armoring of the lower segments because they are not pertinent to this story) comes for therapy because of the general aimlessness of her life and unhappiness in her marriage. In the initial interview, I ask why she had married her husband, and she says that she just drifted into it in the same way that she floats into everything.

In therapy, we have already done some work on the eye segment, and this work has increased her liveliness somewhat; now we are at work on the oral segment. She makes distasteful faces when I suggest that she suck her thumb as she breathes. In the previous sessions she has been willing to suck her thumb for only a few minutes at a time, and rather mechanically; she asks repeatedly to "do something else." In this session, after an initial demurral when I suggest thumb-sucking again, she settles into the pleasure of sucking her thumb, and at one point turns to me to say, "That's not bad." As she continues, she gradually loses herself in the sucking; and as I watch, I note that her respiratory excursions are increasing, which presages a large movement of energy and emotion. She suddenly pulls her thumb from her mouth, coughs several times and erupts into wailing, then sobbing in a bigger voice than I have ever heard from her. When she is finished, she says, "I felt that I wanted M. (her husband) to take care of me completely. You asked me once why I married him, and I didn't know. Now I know."

In psychiatric orgone therapy the emphasis is on work on the biophysical damage that exists in the present. The biophysical block is always the result of traumata from the past, usually from early childhood. We do not engage in long searches into past history. The history often comes to us as the blocks are dissolved. In other cases the armoring yields without the evocation of memories. In some conventional psychotherapies, the patient might have gained an intellectual appreciation of her dependent behavior, but she probably would not have felt it to her marrow as she did when she permitted herself to become a sucking infant. When she went this far, the pain of her position struck her with full force. Then she could stand outside and gain insight into her marriage.

Case 2

A compulsive middle-aged male patient finds it almost impossible to keep his attention on the flashlight I move before his eyes. He constantly distracts himself, clearing his throat with a snort, scratching his face, then his belly, than his scrotum, rubbing his eyes, snorting again, then scratching his head, and so forth. I remonstrate with him to stop all his sideplay and to direct all his attention to following the light. He agrees, follows the light for thirty seconds, and then is off on his wild chase again. This time I begin to mimic him as he goes. When he snorts, I snort; when he scratches, I scratch. He watches me in amusement and says, "I can't keep my mind on the job, heh?" I nod in assent but continue with the imitation. "That's enough," he says, but I persist. "You're a dictator, just like my father," he says half in anger. "I always have to do what somebody else wants me to do."

He has generated enough anger now to be able to focus on the work on eye movement. He moves his eyes now with concentration and diligence and permits himself a level of excitement. The session over, he thanks me and leaves in high spirits.

This is a common type of session in which the superficial layer of defense, the snorting and the scratching, is not permitted to function, forcing the patient to the next deeper level of feeling, anger in this case. Permitting some anger to flow mobilizes energy so that therapeutic work can be accomplished.

Case 3

A forty-year-old male complains of constant weariness and lack of sexual drive, a condition which has persisted for several years. Though he is sensitive and intelligent, he has never made more than a marginal living, working as a store clerk. He is unmarried; and though he finds occasional sexual partners, he never has had a long-term relationship with a woman. In early adolescence he started to have sexual relationships with prostitutes, and he has visited prostitutes periodically throughout his life. The feeling that he's with a "bad" woman adds spice to these encounters. He masturbates compulsively, even after sexual intercourse. In "love-making" he fantasizes constantly. His favorite fantasy is of a menage a trois with a lesbian pair. He has a touching compulsion, is often tortured with obsessions and is aware of pleasure from restraining bowel and bladder evacuation (evidences of strong anality). He is obsequious and submissive. Once in a fight he beat up his opponent and felt guilty for a long time thereafter.

He had been in psychotherapy for several years in childhood and for short periods several times thereafter.

A biophysical examination reveals dull eyes that convey a look of childlike innocence, a thick, unyielding neck and stiff shoulders, a totally flabby abdomen, thin pelvis and spindly legs that look as if they were transplanted from a young adolescent body and are totally disproportionate to the thicker torso.

An early characteristic of his therapy is how quickly he cries. He takes five or ten full breaths, and the tears start flowing, accompanied by childish whimpering. The eyes are capable of nothing but crying. They cannot look angry, tender or frightened. When I request that he make a face, he always draws the muscles toward the center and cries. His reaction to physical pain is the same -- no yell of pain or outrage, only crying. The crying is not full-bodied; it is a step beyond sniveling. His attempts to punch in anger are totally ineffectual. When he tries to kick, he tightens his buttocks, stiffens his spine and moves his legs metronomically.

As a therapist, my problem at this time is whether to attempt first to elicit the deeper crying or the anger, both of which are deeply repressed. Since there are no traces of overt anger, whereas there is a constant display of superficial weeping, I elect to enlarge the crying. With work on the ropes of neck musculature and exhortation to increase the volume of sound, the crying penetrates to farther reaches of the throat and chest until the patient is sobbing. His chest and abdomen are heaving and he makes the palms-upward gesture with his hands to indicate that he is helpless in the face of this onslaught. The sobbing continues at home through the evening. At the next session (the 5th), he says that he had nausea of such severity during the week (the diaphragm is blocking against the tide loosed in the previous visit) that he stayed home from work for several days. Over the next six weeks, he continues to release full-body sobs and we also work on gagging. He is clearly more energetic now and unrealistically (but understandably) optimistic about his future. I warn him against premature optimism, but he ascribes the warning to conservatism on my part. So enthusiastic is he over the therapy that he proselytizes fervently among his friends. I also caution him against this.

He can begin to express some angry affect in his punching now, and he makes menacing faces. On a subsequent visit his breathing produces tingling sensations throughout his trunk and down to his abdomen. This is a new experience; he had formerly felt the sensations only in his hands. He is aware of pleasant genital sensations and strong sexual desire during the following week. After a long hiatus he makes a date with a girl.

In the 24th session he is depressed and drained. He says the bottom dropped out for no apparent reason. As if this weren't enough, he was also nauseated again for several days. His eyes are dead and his voice is weak once again. We return to work on the eyes, but he lacks energy for angry display. In two weeks he is back on the track; anger is more effective than ever, depression is gone, and he reports that his girl likes him.

On the 31st visit he appears shaken. He says that during sexual intercourse he became aware of a strong desire to hurt his girl with his penis. This was tremendously stimulating at first, then so frightening that he became impotent. We do not pursue the discussion of his sexual problem. In the following weeks, he lacks sexual desire and he breaks-off contact with his girl friend.

In the ensuing time, I only repeat the accustomed work on segments down to the diaphragm. I make no attempt to push on because there has been a little more movement than I wish with such a patient.

On the 54th session (approximately one year of therapy) there is the first appearance of diaphragmatic fluttering, a sign that the diaphragmatic block is beginning to give. Sobbing is now even more complete. In recent weeks he has gained in energy, almost to the level of his previous euphoria. On one visit an involuntary spasmodic contraction of the pelvis appears, but I do nothing to encourage its development.

His rage is more potent now. It is reflected in increased independence. He reports pleasant sensations in his pelvis more frequently in therapy (not yet of the tingling variety). He is thinking of starting a small business.

At about the time that he is in therapy for a year and a half, he develops abdominal complaints, such as cramps and occasional diarrhea.

He also develops acute anxiety during a session of merely breathing. He had never experienced anxiety before. His status now is a mixture of positive and negative reactions. On one hand, he is strong, more confident, able to endure more environmental pressure and cognizant of many areas of symptomatic improvement. For example, he no longer has to "work" to achieve a sexual climax. On the other hand, he has more to endure: gastro-intestinal symptoms and occasional anxiety attacks, interlarded with periods of mild depression.

Over the next nine months we work on old segments, clearing the debris that remains after each advance. The gastro-intestinal symptoms become milder and eventually disappear. The anxiety attacks increase in frequency and reach a climax when, in the course of several weeks, the patient has a series of critical dreams. The first is a forthright oedipal dream in which he is having sexual intercourse with his mother. The second is a dream about a household dog from his childhood. In the dream the dog is howling in pain and running from room to room with a bleeding penis. This is a difficult period in therapy. He has panic attacks with fear of dying and often phones me for reassurance. His sexual desire drops to zero, which doesn't distress him at all in view of his other problems.

Over the next months, I keep work on the physical armoring to a minimal, restitutive level. He gradually rises from the state of chronic anxiety to a state of ease and peace. His business is moderately prosperous, his relationship has progressed to the point that he is entertaining thoughts of marriage. In his sexual functioning he no longer fantasizes; he concentrates on the woman instead. His sexual drive is strong and the level of his pleasure is high.

We have done no direct work on his pelvic segment, but neither he nor I have much taste for it. After three-and-a-half years of therapy, he suggests discontinuance, and I agree.

In discussing this patient, I shall forego analysis of the classical psychiatric features of the patient's disorder, which are beyond the projected range of this book, and concentrate on the energetic aspects.

We begin with the physical habitus, which is disproportionate below the torso. There is a well-established principle in biology that form follows function. From what we learn in orgonomy, there is an even earlier principle: both form and function follow the energetic flow. The energy moves out, and the amoeba's pseudopod follows the energetic flow in reaching out to move or to incorporate food. Wherever a patient shows a disproportionate body part (making allowances for birth injuries and genetic factors), there is always a disturbance of function -- but before this, a deficit of energy flow. The people with full bodies and spindly legs, for example, invariably are "unsettled" and unrooted persons, and always have a strong energetic blocking in the lower extremities.

At the beginning of therapy, the patient is a low-energy, ineffectual man with low self-esteem. His sexual energy is at such low ebb that he can perform only with the stimulus of fantasy or the prick of doing a "bad" thing. Even then his energetic discharge is so low that he masturbates afterward. He shows many masochistic features: the pleasure in holding back, then releasing; the simpering; the poor-child look; the obsequious behavior and the low achievement.

The easy tears at the onset of therapy deserve some discussion. Often when the therapist is evaluating the new patient, he asks, "Can you cry?" The patient answers, "Oh yes, I'm crying all the time." This answer does not indicate that the patient is open to his sadness. It usually means that he never reaches to the bottom of his sorrow, that his agony stands intact behind a dam wall, constantly spilling over what the bulkhead cannot contain. The early work with this patient demonstrates that the deeply felt crying is submerged beneath the whimpering.

Efforts to uncover his rage and hate precipitate the premature (from the standpoint of where he is in therapy) display of his sexual sadism. In general, the discoveries come faster and more furiously than one would have desired with this patient. The probable cause of this prematurity is the lack of charge in the patient. He reacts like a bag of gelatin. Once an impulse is set in motion, it keeps going and cannot be contained. One would have preferred that he react more like a sandbag, so that he could better absorb some "punches."

The flabby abdomen is a case in point. Once an impulse was generated through his diaphragm, it tended to reach the pelvis (which had not been sufficiently prepared) directly. Though his abdomen was not tight, it was armored nonetheless, as evidenced by the development of abdominal gastro-intestinal symptoms. The armoring of hypotonicity (lack of tone) is not as well understood as hypertonic armoring. In some cases the impulse passes through a hypotonic area without any hindrance, as it did in this patient, and sometimes the impulse gets lost in a hypotonic area and cannot get through, which is what happens also with fatty armoring.

Though the patient has far more charge at the end of his therapy, the decision to stop at that point is well-considered. Though he has come a long way, he is not the strongest of structures; to proceed further might jeopardize the progress he has achieved. The structure is considered too fragile to open the Pandora's box of the pelvic armoring.

Finally, this case illustrates the ebb and flow of the march through therapy, as contraction succeeds each expansion and is succeeded by the next level of expansion.

Case 4

A woman in her early twenties, typically hysterical in that she always flirts in whatever she does, lies on the coach exhibiting her casual smile, which is part seductive, part "put-on," and withal, a cover for anger. At my request to breathe, she takes two or three full breaths, then launches into chatter. "What do you think of Mann's book on Reich?" I do not answer. "What time is it?" (This is an oft-repeated question, which means that time is passing and we must redouble our efforts to get some meaningful work done.) "I'm a bitch," (which, as an evaluation of the presenting side of her character, is true.) "Do you love me?" (asked semifacetiously). At this juncture I have had enough of this particular defense and I go to work with painful pressure on her armored jaw. She says, "Take off your watch." (The apparent meaning is that as she defends herself against the pressure on her jaw, she may break my watch. On a deeper level, it is a symbolic invitation to undress.) I continue the painful jaw pressure, but deeper. She begins to cry, but soon changes the crying to laughter (bitchiness victorious). I dig into the jaw again and she repeats the request that I take off my watch. Now I pry into her jaw with all my thumb's strength. She says, "Why do you do that when I say, 'take of your watch'?" I answer angrily, "Because you're using it as an excuse for not sticking to the point." She curls up to me, buries her head in my chest and sobs truly. At the point at which I feel her begin to stiffen against the sobbing, I forcible bend her neck back in the position of surrender. She cries deeply and without resistance for the remainder of the hour. When we stop she says, "I felt like calling, 'Mommy.' I never remember calling my mother that."

The simple point of the history of this session is that as a therapist I attacked the array of defenses by a combination of physical assault on the armoring and unmasking of the maneuvering. In this instance the breach was made by my angry exposition of her tricks, but it could not have succeeded without the physical work that preceded it.

Case 5

The patient, a woman in her early forties, is disinclined to work today. Since her eyes are a little out of contact, we begin with breathing and work on eye movement. This work leads to a limited, held kind of crying. I cradle her and the chest begins to heave, releasing fuller, uninhibited crying. Now she is alive through the cervical segment and I begin work on the armored shoulders. I ask her to hit and yell. She answers, "Getting angry involves pitying yourself." I reply, "No, it involves self-respect." She puts effort into the angry expression now, which makes her eyes come even more alive. She asks if we can stop and talk. Because she is vital and serious now, I say, "O.K.."

She tells me that she was feeling well until she walked into the office; then she could feel herself becoming limp, as if a switch were turned-off, and she recognized dependency as a long-standing attention-getter in her life story. Beyond this we discover the anger in "You take care of me." Her release of anger threw the whole mechanism into adult perspective.

Later in the day she calls and says, "I finally got the idea; blessed are the strong."

Case 6

A young college dropout who had worked occasionally as a professional musician complains of "always feeling outside of the action" and of claustrophobia. The "outsider" symptom became acute one year ago under the influence of amphetamines; the claustrophobia developed three months later. With the onset of symptoms, he also had nightmares of his parents' death, of falling in space and of being in a crowd and unable to establish his identity. He feels impelled to be on the move; sitting still makes him nervous. In the past weeks he has been troubled with a steady ringing in his ears. He recognizes a pleasure from scaring people, which he does subtly and sneakily. He always admired the Nazis, but only covertly for fear of social ostracism.

In childhood he was afraid of all kinds of animals and terrified of storms and of his priest, whom he regarded as surrogate God and devil. He was often insomniac; he would be kept awake by visions of infinite space. He wet the bed till age nine or ten. In the family, the mother was the punitive parent and the father was passive. Though he was a "bad" boy, often stealing and indulging in antisocial acts, he identified strongly with Jesus.

He first masturbated at seven or eight with fantasies of pictures from pornographic books. The experience was physically painful. He made sexual overtures to his sister in early adolescence and was rejected. He recalls one clear oedipal dream from childhood. He has a clear memory of witness to a primal scene (parents in sexual intercourse) in childhood.

The medical history was uneventful, except for a familial history of diabetes.

Though he was a precocious student until he attended high school, he associated with the rebellious boys and was always involved in mischief. His current relationships are transitory and chaotic.

Examination on the couch reveals typically schizophrenic "far-off" eyes, with loose armoring through the rest of the body excepting the pelvis. Breathing is very shallow.

When he breathes freely, he perceives strong currents throughout his body, especially in his head and upper extremities. He becomes frightened and begins to tremble. He is soon crying, but there are no tears.

On his next visits he has strongly ambivalent feelings about therapy. He is impressed by the dramatic reactions, but he is mightily scared. During this time I concentrate on mobilizing his chest and working on his eyes. He reveals that sometimes inanimate objects appear to him to be breathing and that object size changes from time to time; he and the objects about him alternately shrink and grow.

In one of the early sessions I make a demonic face and instruct him to express fear with his eyes. In the course of the session, he becomes acutely agitated and reports that he does not see my face but the face of his childhood priest, who had repeatedly threatened him with hell fire. In the following session, he is afraid of me and finds it impossible to look at me. We practice aggression against me with angry faces and pushing against my person. In the first six months we have been focusing on enlivening the chest and eyes and releasing anger. In this time he has existed by scrounging and by leeching on his friends. I deliver an ultimatum -- that within two weeks he must desist from depending on his parents for payment for therapy, or therapy will be discontinued. I assume that now he is capable of self-sufficiency and insist that he employ this potential.

In the following months, he becomes more energetic and increasingly involved with his environment. In his daily life there are instances of spontaneous crying and anger. In our therapeutic work, he feels alive through his torso, but feels nothing below the diaphragm. He develops a block to gazing downward, and soon discovers a conscious fear of looking at the genital region. In one session, we practice focusing on the genitals with the eyes, and it evokes in him strong fears of homosexuality.

As the ability to tolerate the expression of fear in his eyes increases, he becomes more capable of rage, which is expressed against his father and the priest, and against me as their surrogate. At this time (one year in therapy) he has a dream about the priest in which, rather than being terrorized by him, he puts the priest to shame. We have been working on the eyes consistently from the beginning. He is now able to "go off" in his eyes and bring himself back into focused contact at will.

As we begin work on the mouth segment, he obtains more and more gratification from sucking. In an angry outburst after about one-and-a-half years of therapy, he yells, "I want everything, and I want it for nothing!" His infantile dependency is showing.

As awareness of his body increases, he becomes more aware of his bodily clumsiness. We institute a program of creeping and crawling at home, based on the work of Doman and Delacato, who theorize that body coordination develops through stages corresponding to lower, then higher, brain functions. After practicing these exercises for several weeks, he reports a sharpened interest in his environment with (interestingly) more difficulty in walking. With time the walking stability improves.

He is perceiving and enjoying pelvic sensations in therapy now, and in one visit he reports that he "raped" his girlfriend (he didn't rape her, he merely was far more aggressive than usual) and that they both enjoyed it tremendously.

At a little past two years of therapy, his anxiety level increases steadily. In one session there is an orgy of confession in which he reveals, among other things, that he has stolen from his boss and gotten on the welfare rolls though he is still working. Without comment on my part, he discontinues this stealing activity and therapy proceeds.

He is no longer psychotic, but he still has a considerable distance to go toward health. We terminate the story at this juncture because after this point it is not particularly instructive.

The main theme in this case is the long and consistent work on the eyes in the treatment of psychosis. The order of the principal lines of defense in the character analysis is interesting; first, the fear; then the rage; beneath that a layer of submission and dependency which relates to yet another fear, that of homosexuality. Of additional interest is the reversion to an old defensive pattern (stealing) when threatened by the developing pelvic anxiety.

Chapter 9
The Therapist

The Taoists have a saying: "When the wrong man uses the right means, the right means works in the wrong way." In accordance with this principle, there is a concerted effort in orgonomy to insure that the "right" man is in charge of the means. In the United States every orgonomist must be a physician. This requirement is established because, though some psychologists are competent to deal with the psychological aspects of therapy, medical training is considered essential to understanding and treating the body as one does in medical orgonomy. Moreover, the aspiring therapist is required to obtain certification in his specialty (usually psychiatry, but certification in internal medicine or obstetrics, for example, is acceptable when the therapist's orgonomic interests lie in these directions). Certification is required to assure classical competence in the field. In addition, the aspiring orgonomist must be trained for several years in didactic course work, laboratory courses, seminars, and supervised therapy before he is considered ready to treat patients.

The therapist must reach an established level of biophysical freedom in his own structure before he is permitted to treat patients orgonomically. The most important prerequisite is the stability of the therapist's character structure and his ability to pulsate freely and to feel and express his full range of emotions without anxiety. He attains this first, through whatever good fortune in childhood kept him relatively alive emotionally, and then through his own therapy, which unties his knots.

In orgonomic work, competence and health vary from time to time. Each of us carries the hidden traces of his sickness. It is presumed that the therapist has reached that state of perception in which he can recognize his sickness if and when it reappears. If it is only mild, he must be aware of it in his dealings with his patients. If it is severe, he should withdraw from professional contact with his patients until he has recovered. I am not speaking here of such sickness as psychotic breakdown, but of the emergence of character traits that do damage to patients.

If, for example, personal anxiety should temporarily prevent the therapist from being able to admit that in a given situation he is wrong, or from understanding what is going on, then he stands in the way of his patients' growth and development. Or if he fails to come down on a patient who is abusing the therapeutic situation, he is failing the patient again.

The patient often attributes magical virtues to the therapist and can be disappointed, and sometimes vengeful, when he discovers the therapist's feet of clay. The therapist is supposed to never get sick, to always be happy, to have the perfect family. There is a certain logic to this expectation. The therapist who is constantly sick, who is living in a bored, inert marriage would certainly be suspect; but the perfection that the patient seeks is often unreasonable.

Though the therapist should be energetic enough to keep the treatment alive and moving, some days he feels that there is a boiled onion where his brain should be. He does not see what there is to be seen; he feels nothing. On such days he would be a boring companion, let alone therapist. On these days he plods mechanically through his work, rousing himself as much as possible. Something is accomplished at such times by patients who are already moving and no longer depend on his energy. For the others, not much may be achieved except that they learn that sometimes the therapist is as dead as they.

On other days, the therapist's perception crackles. With each succeeding patient, he sees little subtle aspects of the body armoring or behavior that he missed for months. These exhilarating days neutralize those times when, after three depressed patients in a row, the therapist feels as if the life has been blotted out of him. On these unusually good days, the contact with patients is mutually enlivening.

There are other times when the therapist is especially sensitive to armoring in a particular segment. This is probably a reflection of unusual vitality of that segment of his own body at that time.

In spite of the high's and low's of his energy system, the therapist must have a steady sufficiency of energy over the long period in order to conduct therapy successfully. His energy and stability tides him and his patients over the times when he adds two and two and concludes that the sum is five; when he is grouchy and unreasonable; when he forgets what the patient has already told him; and when he inflicts his enthusiasms and his prejudices onto his patients.

Because the therapeutic technique is potent, it carries the potential for great harm as well as good. There are heady adventurists in the psychotherapeutic professions who, untrained, have "borrowed" from Reich and injured their patients, physically and emotionally. With a technique that can be physically painful, there must be assurance that the therapist has no hidden characterologic reason to hurt. In a therapy involving physical as well as deep emotional contact, in which sexual energies are freed, the patient must be insured against the abuse of the professional relationship. Reich was strict in this matter. He recommended that any therapist who, because of life circumstance, was temporarily unfulfilled sexually should withdraw from conducting therapy with members of the opposite sex until the problem was solved.

The therapist's basic character structure will show in his work with patients. There are "tough" therapists who conduct therapy in a predatory fashion: they are especially helpful to patients with a bag of sneaky tricks. And there are more paternal (or maternal) therapists who establish contact with patients with long histories of abuse. In the course of his own therapy, each therapist should have uncovered enough of his own soft self to be sensitive to the delicate qualities of his patient, and enough of his own aggression to pursue his patients' defenses rigorously.

Contrary to many patients' expectations, the therapist is not a paragon of health. Somewhere there are persons who, by virtue of genetic endowment, rare, straight and sensible parents and smiling fates, have never heard of Reich or orgonomy, but who have achieved a natural level of health beyond that of the therapist. And every experienced therapist knows that some of his patients have achieved a fuller level of health than he. No matter; perfection is not a qualification for conducting useful therapy. A sufficient characterologic restructuring and a comprehensive education in understanding the disease processes guarantee that the orgonomist will be a decent and thoughtful guide to the misguided.

The therapist is obliged to keep his own house in order. If he pussy-foots in any aspect of his life, his work with patients will eventually bear traces of pussy-footedness. Like his patients, he should exercise regularly and provide adequately for play, vacation and the pursuit of other interests so that he can be continually renewed. He must always be on guard against the reappearance of his own armoring and take adequate measures against it when it occurs. He must maintain his contact with nature so that he can distinguish between the real and the assumed.

Chapter 10
Self-Regulation in Children

In the course of their therapy patients are sometimes requested to gather their childhood photographs and bring them in for inspection. In this way we can often witness the specific time period in which particular armoring had its onset. One sees the eyes open and bright up to a specific time, then a photograph with veiled eyes, and the consistent dulled eyes thereafter. Sometimes, when the circumstances of the critical period are discussed, it is possible to reconstruct the cause and effect patterns.

The significant armoring is always laid down in childhood. Knowledge of this has several uses. If I am assured that my childhood environment shaped me, let's say, to irresponsibility, ineptness and hatred, I can use the knowledge to torture my parents, bemoan my fate, throw up my hands when called to task. In short, I can employ it to defend the continuance of my sickness. Or, if I am serious, I can employ my energies in eradicating my defeats, whose history I now know; and most important, I can be forewarned of my potential for harming my child.

When I observe my cat delivering her kittens, I am amazed at her instinct and her efficiency in mothering. I have no apprehension that (barring human interference) lionesses will not raise their cubs effectively to lionhood or that alligator mothers will not raise their babies correctly. I have every apprehension about human mothers and human babies in our society. Whereas my cat knows how to conduct her parturition and how to minister to her litter, my patients and friends and their advisors -- their mothers, aunts, neighbors and doctors -- do not. The reason is simple. My cat is one with her nature; the humans have renounced their nature and have suffered armoring in its stead.

Children's environments are peopled with anxious mothers, bland mothers, "model" mothers, harassed mothers, loving mothers, harried fathers, jealous fathers, irritable fathers, boozy fathers, caring fathers, parents who battle for dominance, ignore one another, tolerate one another, contradict one another, are considering separating from one another, or genuinely care for one another. The cast of characters is integral to the story line. In the nuclear family setting, the mother is usually the more important parent in the earliest years, whether because there is a special bonding that results from carrying and delivering her child or because of her more constant presence in caring for the child. There is a general fantasy that every mother is uniquely equipped to raise her child. The state of humankind is the sorry answer to that dream. Most mothers, warped by their warped mothers, trapped by their structures, are means to warp their children. Most mothers and most fathers are benumbed parents. Genuine maternal love -- love that implies healthy contact with the needs and moods of the child -- is a rare phenomenon.

In most cases, child-rearing is not a process of nurturing the nature that unfolds in the child, but of molding the personality of the child until it conforms to the parents' needs. When we are consistently considerate of his purpose we naturally educate the child to behave considerately. Armored parents teach the artifice of mannerly behavior by precept. A healthy parent regards the fulfillment of the child's needs in early infancy as more important than the satisfaction of her own. She is able to function in this manner because she is not burdened by unsatisfied infantile needs that conflict with those of her child. As the child grows past infancy, the balance of child vs. parental need shifts toward equality. The parent occasionally denies the child to satisfy her own immediate need. Providing that the child's essential requirements were cared for, the establishment of the parent's needs as equal in importance to the child's enables the child to become reasonable in his demands and to respect others' rights.

The armored parent regards her need as infinitely more significant than the child's. She rules by edict and establishes separate standards of conduct for herself and her child. She demands of the child, "Why did you do that?" Armored parents mold children -- that is, they demand conformity at the expense of armoring. The molding process takes place at the cost of the child's spontaneity. Conformity can only be bought and paid for at the price of becoming dead somewhere, somewhere distorted. This is not high-flown orgonomic theory. The process was observed decades ago by Margaret Ribble,[16] independent of Reich's influence.

The problem of molding children in the armored parental image is at the root of the problem of a sick humanity. Warping the structure of what Reich called "the highly plastic bio-energy system" of the

[16] Ribble, M. *Infantile Experience in Relation to Personality Development, in Personality and the Behavior Disorders*, J. McV. Hunt, N.Y., 1944.

young child can be accomplished with remarkable ease. Reich[17] reported on the armoring of a five-week-old infant whose mother was rated "fairly healthy" by observers of the orgonomic Infant Research Center. If an infant born to parents who are sentient of the dangers of armoring falls victim in five weeks, it is no wonder that in practice one meets an eight-year-old suffering from behavior and speech problems with a chest almost rigid as wood. When one meets such a child, the question fairly screams in one's head: "Is such extensive damage really necessary to raise children to adulthood?"

When Freud discovered the natural history of the psychosexual development of infants and children, he documented what, to that time, was the most scientific revolution of how nature works to make a child a man. Yet even he, entrapped by his own armoring, was forced to deny the implications of his discovery and, instead, to rationalize in support of emotional repression. Confusing the unconscious of armored man with the core of unrepressed man, he reasoned that a failure of repression would lead to barbarity. The child's free, natural flow must be restrained, he thought, to control the savage in man.

Given the advantage of orgonomic insight and the opportunity to observe some children grown through adolescence free of significant repression (armoring), neither savage nor uncivilized, but bright and social and sweet, I find Freud's intellectual arguments empty. In his defense it must be said that, where armoring exists, defense against it is necessary for the societal welfare.

Man is born neither in "sin" nor, as the mystics would have it, in a state of grace. He is born, as all animals, with energies, instincts and a genetic physical-chemical program for development and maturation. The distortions in thinking that armoring imposes have caused us, on one hand, to raise children by "training" them out of the "original sin" which we assumed and, on the other hand, to neglect their basic needs. Inattention leads to armoring as surely as molding. The human infant depends on the devoted maternal response for its fulfillment. Failing this, it is frustrated; and frustration leads to armoring. The mother who has lost the desire to breast-feed her baby and the mother who gives facetious answers to her child's serious questions are failing to bring out their children's reactive potential. Their children will be less complete than they could be.

---

[17] Reich, W., "Armoring in a Newborn Infant," *Orgone Energy Bulletin*, Vol. 3, July, 1951.

Reich saw the frustrating and distorting mechanisms of child-rearing practices with a crystal vision. As a scientist, he saw that the armored child was a twisted child. As an observer of the human scene, he noted that something inherently terrible was happening to the human spirit as it grew from child to man.

For readers interested in the subject of how parents armor their children, I would recommend The Agony in the Kindergarten [18](unfortunately out of print, but perhaps the library has a copy).

There is no unarmored child, nor any unarmored adult. Even in the best case, the child who is raised by relatively healthy parents is subjected to a host of social pressures that infringe upon his ability to be himself fully. We do not know what an unarmored human would be. To find the answer, Reich founded the Orgonomic Infant Research Center (OIRC) whose purpose was to focus on the social influences that lead to armoring of children, to observe and describe unarmored infants, and so far as possible to function as a body that fights for the rights of children to be true to their own natures. In the OIRC, a half dozen trained workers made detailed observations of a mother through her pregnancy and delivery and followed the growth of her child for months after birth. The staffing may seem excessive to the reader, but we were treading in unknown territory and one pair of vigilant eyes might have discerned what another had missed. The OIRC no longer functions, but every practicing orgonomist carries on the work in some little way.

Reich's guiding principle for parenting is self-regulation. Self-regulation does not equal laissez faire; that is the practice of lazy, uncaring, contactless mothers. Self-regulation is not related either to permissiveness or discipline. It means being alive to the child's needs for nurture, both physical and emotional, and to his need for stimulation and education; above all, it means supporting the child's individuality. The self-regulated child chooses his activities so far as he is capable. When he is unhappy he is permitted to cry; he is comforted, but his crying is not smothered or distracted. His anger is accepted. His love is returned. His fears are recognized and alleviated when possible. When he acts to hurt himself or others, the parent corrects him to the limit of his understanding. When, at age one, he tears pages from the book his mother is reading, she moves books out of his reach. When, at age five, he tears pages from her book, her anger convinces him that he must not

---

[18] Steig, M., *The Agony In The Kindergarten*, Dueli, Sloan and Pearce, N.Y., 1950.

do that again. In short, he's taught to distinguish between freedom and license.

Relatives who constantly tickle him or encourage him to smile in an unwitting attempt to shape him in their vapid pleasantness are instructed that he does not always have to smile or be pleasant. Sometimes he prefers to sit quietly and examine them (which makes them anxious), or not pay attention to them, or frown or scowl, or be dopey. Anyone who tells him that he's a "bad" boy for having committed some infantile act is banished. When he is a small child, anyone who berates him for not sharing is given a sermon on the failure of their altruism toward him. No one is permitted to foist their notions of good behavior on him. He is treated with respect, and that is how he learns respect. When he is at the age of understanding, he is taught -- as he "tests the limits" of acceptable behavior -- that he has no right to infringe on others' freedom, just as they have no right to infringe on his. Sometimes his and others' rights will collide, and he will learn the art of accommodation.

If there is a tendency in society to pathogenicity which infects the character structure of infants and children, and if, at least theoretically, this is a society based on law and justice, then there are no laws more necessary for society and, indeed, the world than those for the protection of newborns and children. In 1952 Reich proposed such laws to the Congressional Committee on Foundations.[19] He noted that there were no laws that forbade infringing upon the child's natural rights. This may sound exaggerated, but remember that even laws protecting the battered child have been promulgated only in recent decades. Charles Lowe[20] is among those who have noted this failure of the law.

---

[19] Reich, W., "On Laws Needed for the Protection of Life in Newborns and of Truth," *Orgone Energy bulletin,* Vol. V, March, Nos. 142 and 143, 1953.

[20] Lowe, Charles, M.D., "Child Care," *Science and Public Policy*, Vol. 4, No. 1, January 1968.
"I would therefore propose that a single agency be established with a director of cabinet rank to deal with all federal services and research related to children.

[1]   The child has no spokesman in government. We have a cabinet post for transportation and for our national parks. Do we lack the vision or wisdom to create an equal post for the benefit of our most valuable national resource?

[2]   Child care must be viewed not as a sentimental whim of the public, but rather as an overwhelmingly important constituent of our culture. Effective planning or research on, and service for children demands that there be created within the government a unique position with administrative strength and powerful political leverage. If the incumbent in such a position ... combines compassion with vision, articulates effectively, and plans soundly, we may yet rescue our children and prepare them for the future."

This call for laws protecting newborns and children is in line with Reich's view of society as the patient. He saw the futility of treating emotionally disturbed children and adults, solving each instance of spoilage perpetrated by armored men, while the process of armoring children proceeds in perpetuity.

Reich was no wild-eyed visionary. He did not expect that his call would alert society to this truth, that parents will turn about and raise their children rationally, and that in one or two generations the "new man" would emerge. Reich spoke in terms of many, many generations and hundreds of years before the "children of the future" would emerge in significant numbers.

But now we are enlightened by his vision, and we can make a beginning. He said, "We cannot tell our children what kind of world they will or should build. But we can equip our children with the kind of character structure and biological vigor which will enable them to make their own decisions, to find their own ways, to build their own future and that of their children, in a rational manner."[21] If there were a hundred times as many therapists as practice currently, the number of people affected by the therapeutic process would still be statistically negligible. For this reason, Reich often said that the orgonomist whose activity was confined exclusively to private practice was not worthy of the name. In a sick world, therapists' dedication had to be larger than helping a few sick individuals toward health.

It is imperative that the orgonomist fill the spaces left in Reich's pioneering scientific discoveries and ultimately extend these insights, that he rests on the problems of society and its institutions in the light of his awakened discernment and, above all, that he help protect the future of humanity by making what inroads he can on the processes of child-rearing that perpetuate the human sickness.

Infant research has been a keystone of orgonomic scientific investigation. With Aries,[22] Reich assumes that we have been blind to the child's needs. Our communications with newborns, infants and children are largely arrogant and unfeeling broadcasts; we are not tuned to receiving messages. Consequently, we know almost nothing about infants that could not be obtained by mechanistic data-gathering.

The entire field of medical and parental practices with regard to the newborn and infant has to be reexamined. How much of what we do

---

[21] Reich, W., "Children of the Future," *Orgone Energy Bulletin,* Vol. 2, No. 4, October, 1959.
[22] Aries, P., *Centuries of Childhood*, Alfred A. Knapf, 1962.

to the infant and expect of him is in blind conformity to the medical texts, the state laws, the expectations of our own mothers and aunts, our religion, our need for approval? To what extent was our interaction with our children a simple and direct reaction, a respectful response to their needs?

Consider, for example, feeding practices in the typical American hospital[23]. Infants are fed on schedules, typically four-hour schedules. Is this because new borns get hungry every four hours? To find the answer, we must observe healthy babies who are on demand feeding. After observing a number of these, we see that the four-hour figure is a maternity ward mystique. The infant who eats at his own discretion may take the breast for a half hour, then desire it again in an hour and suck for ten minutes, then sleep for 6 or 8 hours. The four-hour designation has no relation to the infant's needs; it is predicated on the convenience and efficiency of hospital personnel.

The new mother who has been awaiting her child and has made plans for its comfort assumes that the doctors and nurses will aid her in this endeavor. When they tell her to feed her baby at four-hour intervals, she does their bidding because theirs is informed authority. She is not aware that the doctors and nurses are deaf to her baby's voice. She does not know that in this instance the needs of the institution take precedence over the needs of the baby.

The child's problems with the world may have had their onset long before his arrival in the delivery room. Cultural superstitions, financial worries, a callous or brutal husband, her own neurotic structure may have caused the expectant mother to carry her baby through pregnancy in a uterus that was contracted with anxiety. Long before actual birth the environment could have been exerting harmful influences upon the growing fetus. We know, for example, that there is a correlation between increased fetal heart rate and the incidence of anxious states in later life, though we do not yet have many solid studies in this area. The scientific knowledge of the functional aspects of the intrauterine environment and its effect on the fetus is in its infancy. Obviously, all noxious influences cannot be abolished, but we must be sentient to the rights of the fetus and aware that his environment should be an optimal one.

---

[23] In recent years there has been notable improvement with more freedom for mother-neonate contact, but often the institutional convenience takes precedence over the infant's needs.

One cannot speak of the desirability of a pleasurable pregnancy and a relaxed uterus without handling the problem of the mother's character structure and, beyond that, the disturbing influences of her immediate environment and the social institutions which shape her. If her religion implies that she must pay for the sin of sexual gratification by bearing her child in pain, then we who espouse the cause of the unborn child must challenge her religious belief and instruct her in ways to bear her child with a minimum of pain and in contact with the joy of childbirth.

So far as possible, we attempt to decrease the intensity of the mother's armoring during her pregnancy. A free chest increases the oxygenation of the blood of mother and baby, augments the mother's energy level, enables her to function more freely emotionally and will be an aid in the expeditious birth of her child. Clearing armoring in the eye segment will help her to go through parturition alive to the miracle of the process and ready to greet her child. Above all, we attempt to loosen the lower segments, particularly the pelvic segment, so that the pelvis will not contract about the fetus during pregnancy nor hinder the birth process at delivery. In several deliveries performed under orgonomic auspices, the obstetrician attended to the actual delivery of the child and the orgonomist kept watch against any tendency to armor, particularly in the eyes. This function need not be performed by a therapist but could be done by a husband or friend or any informed, relatively unarmored person with whom the mother can establish good contact.

Whenever possible, mothers are encouraged to bear their children naturally. Where this is not possible, local anesthesia such as caudal block is infinitely preferable to a general anesthetic, which anesthetizes both child and mother and makes birth a process from which both have to "recover." The local anesthetic relieves the mother of her pain while enabling her to be at least a partial witness (her anesthetized pelvis is not a witness) to her child's entry into the world; and she is present to welcome him. We decry the use of obstetrical stirrups. What an upside-down system that delivers babies uphill, against gravity!

Following birth, the infant should not be fussed with by medical personnel with a compulsive itch to make him clean and sterile. He should be placed in his mother's arms, next to her breast, and the two can, at long last, meet.

This is the point at which modern obstetrical and pediatric practice often enter to institute a process of dehumanization of both mother and child. Silver nitrate is often instilled into the child's eyes[24], mucus is aspirated from the mouth and sometimes gauze is applied (often unnecessarily roughly) to collect excess mucus. The child is cleansed and dispatched to the nursery to cry with the other nursery babies. A variable period of separation of mother and child ensues until the hospital or pediatrician's protocol determines that mother and child may reunite for a feeding.

Silver nitrate is a caustic solution that is instilled into the newborn's eyes to kill any gonococci that the baby may have picked up in the birth canal, and that may later cause a gonorrheal infection of the eye and, possibly, blindness. State law generally decrees that either silver nitrate or an antibiotic be applied to newborns' eyes to forestall this possibility. The silver nitrate is an irritant and within a few days many infants develop purulent eye infection from the caustic solution. Antibiotics are not caustic, and if chosen judiciously, they also destroy gonococci. The problem with the antibiotic is that in very rare cases it can cause a sensitization reaction. Orgonomists oppose the use of silver nitrate because the infant, instead of experiencing the world freshly, with warmth and comfort, is immediately exposed to a painful insult to his eyes that must interfere with his earliest eye contact with his mother. Certainly where the possibility of gonorrheal infection exists the infant must be protected. But why must every newborn be traumatized? It is apparent to obstetricians that the majority of delivering females are not gonorrheic. Their babies should have no eye instillations. Where gonorrhea is suspect in the mother, or where a positive diagnosis has been established, an antibiotic should be instilled, permitting the newborn to maintain relatively free eye contact.

The significance of early eye contact was largely overlooked before Reich. The armoring of the eye segment in the earliest weeks and its relationship to the later development of schizophrenia, "idiopathic" epilepsy, depersonalization and other disorders has been well established in medical orgonomy.

Another medical practice very widely performed in American hospitals and decried in orgonomy is the routine circumcision of male newborns. For a detailed argument of the medical propositions for and

---

[24] Antibiotics are used or this purpose in recent years.

against routine circumcision, the reader is referred to Gardner,[25] Herskowitz,[26] and Preston.[27] From a purely medical point of view, there are as many good reasons for not performing circumcision as there are for performing it. Spock[28] understands this but still recommends it because, since most other boys have been circumcised, circumcision of this child will help make him feel "regular." Pursuing this logic, one assumes that if Spock were practicing in an area where tribesmen regularly circumcised clitorises (as they do, for example, in some parts of Africa) he would assist in the practice to help the girls feel "regular." One expects that, in medical matters, practitioners should lead society rather than follow social customs.

From an orgonomic view, the practice of infant circumcision is savage. A painful operation (and it is painful) performed on the genitals of the child newly arrived in he world is essentially a reflection of man's sexual sickness. The root reasons for the performance of the operation reach to deeper emotional levels than the alleged medical excuses.

Let us now return to the problem of the newborn removed to the nursery. The reasons offered for the infant's transference are: 1) the mother has gone through a traumatic time; she needs rest; 2) the breasts do not yet contain milk, only nonnutritive colostrum; 3) we do not want to overburden the baby's kidneys; 4) the child will sleep, anyway, and be unaware of where he is. 5) Unstated, but high in the consideration of the hospital personnel, is the preoccupation with antisepsis and sterility. The mother's environs are viewed as germy and the nursery as sterile. The frequency with which hospital nurseries are quarantined has done nothing to dislodge this prejudice.

It is true that the mother often needs a rest following delivery. This is as much a function of her armored organism and the unnatural procedures to which she has been subjected as to anything pertaining to parturition per se. The healthy mother reports that as soon as her child is in her arms, sucking at her breast, there is a marvelous amnesia that sets in concerning the discomfort she endured in the birthing process. It

[25] Gardner, D., "The Fate of the Foreskin," *British Medical Journal,* Vol. 12, pages 1433 -- 1437.

[26] Hertzkowitz, M., "The Mechanistic Distortion of Treatment of Infants and Children," *Journal of American College of Neuropsychiatrists,* No. 3, pages 13 -- 18, 196?

[27] Preston, "Whither the Foreskin, *JAMA,* Vol. 213, No. 11, September 14, 1970.

[28] Spock, B., *The Common Sense Book of Baby and Child Care,* Duell, Sloan, and Pearce, N.Y., 1945.

is as if a page had been turned and now she is caught up in her new experience.

Anyone who has witnessed the birth of puppies or kittens will recall that the mother immediately licks the infant, establishing contact, and lifts it to a teat where it sucks. The unnaturalness of removal to a nursery is revealed in an experiment by Lee Salk in which he broadcast a mother's heartbeat into a nursery and very significantly reduced the level of crying and fretting; he also noted a significant weight gain in the babies who received the broadcast as compared to controls -- despite the same food intake.

It is true that the mother's breast is not filled with nutritive milk at first, but the infant's sucking is the best stimulus for the flow of milk. The immediate sucking of the newborn effects a physiological reflex in the mother that causes her uterus to clamp down to decrease post-partum bleeding. Obstetricians administer a hormone by injection to accomplish this for mothers separated from their babies. The colostrum has a beneficial, slightly laxative effect on the infant. But the comparison of the rosy, freely breathing suckling newborn with his paler, fretful counterpart in the nursery is the most telling argument. Before 1944, Margaret Ribble had noted in her study of 600 newborn infants that those who had been separated from their mothers exhibited perceptible muscular tension, breathing irregularities and feeding problems. She noted that the tensions tended to persist and become a kind of "primitive anxiety."

There is abundant evidence to indicate that infants put to breast following birth and put on demand feeding lose less weight in the first days, and are subsequently healthier and happier than separated and scheduled infants.

The infant fed on schedule is a frustrated infant. His natural timetable is being thwarted. The demand-fed infant has a feeling of security and experiences the new world as a place where his needs are satisfied. The healthy mother regulates her life at this time to meet her child's needs. The armored mother minds the clock rather than her baby. It is no wonder, then, that the most profound emotional disorders, the psychoses, have roots in these earliest days[29] when the world can be experienced so diversely; from pleasantly stimulating and fulfilling to hostile, boring, uncaring and frustrating.

---

[29] There are other roots to psychoses, e.g. genetic, but the environmental ones are those we can do something about.

152

The orgonomist views the child's development throughout the psychosexual stages from the perspective of fulfillment of his requirements. The development of armoring is taken as a sign that something has gone awry.

From birth, the healthy mother engages her child's eyes whenever possible. She speaks with her eyes as much as she is able, and he learns to speak with his. The environment abounds with colors, shapes, movement to encourage lively vision.

Breast-feeding of the infant is preferred over bottle feeding. Mother's milk is the most complete infant food. Breast-feeding allows the establishment of a natural bond between mother and child. In those instances, however, where a mother is temperamentally set against breast-feeding, the infant will be best served if it is bottle-fed. The infant will sense that the mother was coerced to breast-feed against her inclination and will react with distress.

Breast-feeding should be continued for as long as it is mutually pleasurable to mother and child. The mouthing needs are not satisfied in a year, as is attested by the thumb-suckers, smokers, chewers, nail-biters and nonstop talkers. If breast-feeding must be terminated before the infant's sucking needs are fully satisfied, the bottle should be substituted for as long as the child desires.

A mother who was cognizant of her child's oral needs made arrangement with the teachers for her child to take her bottle to nursery school at age four. Because the school was "free," the teachers acquiesced, though with nervous smiles. The child sucked her bottle at rest periods for three or four days and then (because of the teacher's anxiety), she stopped. However, she continued to take her bottle at bedtime until she was almost six. Children who stayed overnight would have an invariable response. They would say, "You still take a bottle? Only babies take bottles." To which she would reply, "Oh, no I'm not a baby, I just like a bottle when I go to bed."

By the second, or certainly the third overnight stay, the young visitors would ask her mother, "Can I have a bottle, too, when I go to bed?"

The ministrations of cultist parents can be discerned at all levels of the child's psychosexual development. The cultist "buys" an "enlightened" view of child-rearing though he lacks the emotional solvency with which to make the purchase. His understanding of the matter is purely intellectual, so it is a misunderstanding. He cannot raise a free child, though his child wears a badge proclaiming, "I am free."

A five-year-old boy ran into the house from his ball game in the street. His mother was conversing with a friend. While they talked, he fumbled at her blouse, extracted a breast, took a quick squirt, shoved the breast away and ran out to his friends to play.

The interchange has no relevance to oral needs though it was an endpoint of a cultist principle that the child must never be frustrated orally. The message in that meeting spoke of a problem more serious than oral frustration. The child's act spoke of disdain and a need to stop the foolishness. It said, "Here is absurd behavior in payment for your duplicity."

The ocular and oral stages are concurrent at the beginning of life, and fashion the child's basic attitudes toward the world and his place in it. The ocular development determines how he sees the world, whether he reaches out to meet and discover it, or whether he retreats into himself from it. If the child lacks pleasant, interesting, secure stimulation in the first weeks and months, that lack of stimulation will affect his integration, openness, liveliness and interest. This kind of deprivation may cause him later in life to be unable to pursue tasks to their completion or to concentrate.

It used to be alleged that newborn infants do not see. Some older physicians, uneducated to recent studies, still maintain it. However, the facts speak otherwise. We not only know that newborns see, we can even measure their visual acuity and what sights interest them most. What we are unable to measure is the special quality of the healthy infant's gaze. The intense concentration, the purity of that way of looking is preserved in only a special few of us as we grow into life.

Orality complements the eye function in helping the child determine a root identity and establish an original fix on himself in a universe of others. The mouth is the way we first experience that there is "me" and there is something outside of me that either lovingly supplies me with what I desire or pays no or little attention to me. In the best case, that "other" will be an individual with a strong, clearly delineated energy field, a person to reckon with; in the worst, an individual with a weak, diffuse field, sans "presence," ineffectual.

The anal stage of psychosexual development is an artifact of culture. Whereas the oral and the genital stages are natural and inevitable, the anal stage is hinged to a social act -- toilet training. If

154

there were no attempt to train the child, no preoccupation with bowel and bladder functions, there would be no anal stage and no anal character traits.

Ideally children should be left to train themselves. If the home is sensible and stable, children toilet-train themselves by three or four. However, a mother who has her own problems concerning excretory functions, whether soiled diapers are extremely distasteful to her, or the fact that the neighbor's child is trained at this age makes her anxious, or she lacks the conviction to face her mother's criticism, it would be better for her child to be trained. She should start as late as possible and never use pressure or shame or punishment -- only praise for successful learning, understanding for mistakes, and patience.

The child who is trained, no matter how patiently, will have learned to be preoccupied with excretory functions for months of his childhood, and will lack the security of the self-regulated child who wanted to do something that was more grown-up and achieved it by himself.

The child who is trained too early and too severely (I once saw psychotic twins who had been toilet-trained by six months) is bent to do what others want, irrespective of his understanding of the need or his willingness to accede. His focus henceforth is that he must do what "they" want; what he wants is of less importance. He becomes tight with the rage that he must repress at this violation of his nature. Superficially he is compliant. Rigidity is his hallmark, perfection his goal. He can never experiment, never stray. He never gets to live his life.

The healthy mother may lift her valuable rugs from the floor until her child has attained sphincter control. Her child may sometimes be diapered, but at times she will allow him to enjoy going unclothed, and rather than project her anxiety about soiled rugs onto her child, she will forego their pleasure temporarily. Or she may keep them down and clean them as best she can. She will try to keep her cleanliness needs from impinging on her child's need to grow free.

The cultist (who has attained enlightenment, but lacks sense) announces to the assembled Saturday evening company in his four-year-old daughter's presence that the newspaper-strewn floor is for his daughter to make kaka whenever she wants.

He may also permit his pets to defecate where they will, mistaking the toilet smells for a state of nature. He has so little contact with nature that he never learned that animals don't foul their nests.

The child who is self-regulated will not be prone to compulsive rigidity, acquisitiveness, sadism, miserliness, characterologic passive resistance, enuresis (bedwetting), constipation, hemorrhoids and other lower bowel syndromes. The dirt that crusts the earth will still be handled with pleasure. The child will never need to tell or laugh at toilet jokes to dispel his anal anxiety. His buttocks, thighs and sphincters will not be held in a state of chronic contraction that will attenuate his sexual pleasure.

As children grow to the genital stage, they come with varying fractions of the energy they were born with. The children crippled severely in the pregenital phases arrive at the gates of genitality already dulled and devitalized. More fortunate children come with the bounty of their vigorous young energy and savor the newly intensified genital pleasures. But if they now come into conflict with the genital anxiety of their parents, it is these more lively children who suffer the most acute genital frustration.

It is an axiom of therapy that there is no anxiety to compare with the anxiety released when the pelvic armoring is approached. The facile intellectual play with sexual overtones and the various sexual atheleticisms are clearly revealed as defensive maneuvers when the sexual libertarian and the sexual athlete meet their pelvic anxiety and run in dismay. The repressed ascetic is not unique in his fear of sexual pleasure.

The outrage of the parent who discovers his little girl in sexual play with the neighbor boy or the firm admonition, "Never let me catch you doing that again," when the child is discovered fondling his genitals are not the only traumata of the genital stage.

"I always hated the way my mother wiped my face. It was always rough, and I knew it meant she didn't like me. I can even remember when she changed my diapers and it was the same thing. The feeling I got was that I was a pain in the neck. And both kinds of wiping left a certain feeling under my skin. Then when I was ten or eleven, I started to get this buzzing in my scrotum and testicles, and it felt kind of nice. I asked my mother what it was, and I don't remember exactly what she said but the meaning was "buzz off." It gave me the same kind of feeling I got when she would wipe me. I gradually learned to keep that feeling down, then finally I didn't feel it anymore."

The signal may be subtle -- avoidance of touching certain parts of the body while bathing the child, glancing away from genital areas when the child is undressed, distracting the child with conversation or play whenever his hands move toward his genitals. And there are the provocative signals of other sexually sick parents -- the thinly veiled excuses to ogle the stimulating sexual parts by voyeuristic adults, the seductive fondling and parading by sexually unsatisfied parents. Just as the orally blocked mother transmits her oral disease to her child, and the anally injured parents convey their sick anal messages to their children, sexually distorted parents bestow their problem sexuality upon their children.

The cultist at this stage of the child's development makes a point of his nudity in the child's presence and invites the child to witness the sexual intercourse of his parents. There is nothing implicitly harmful in the casual and comfortable nudity of parents and children. The danger lies in the fact that what is essentially simple and natural has, with us, taken on complicated and twisted overtones. The sweet air is rarely sweet within us or without us anymore.

Parents who make their child audience to their love-making have become unnatural. They are insensitive to the fact that the lumination of the two superimposed energy fields in genital embrace is diminished and distorted by the presence of another energy field. Beyond this, they demean the experience of loving in favor of sex as entertainment or "instruction." We have lived with the fallacy of the witness of the primal scene as an invariable super trauma to the child's psyche. The fact that Samoans grow up in a single room where they witness the lovemaking of their parents and sisters many nights over, yet grow to adulthood less emotionally disturbed than we, belies the implicit trauma of primal scenes. It is not the witness of the primal scene per se that is traumatizing; it is the guilt and sexual sickness with which the scene is charged. Now we are entering the time of the opposite fallacy -- of the primal scene as instruction laboratory.

If there has not been significant damage in the pregenital stages, genitality requires no nudging. The body's own energy is quite sufficient for healthy sexual growth, barring interference. Between the Scylla of parental avoidance and Charybdis of parental meddling lies the natural route of the child's pleasurable experience of genital flow --

the direct, honest, parental answers to questions, the child's experimentation that follows, and his development in his own way. A patient remembering the deep and gentle sexual longing for a girlfriend when he was a little boy said, "Someday somebody who has a clear line to these memories, because he didn't have to repress them, will write a book called The Sensuous Child."

The child blocked at the oral or anal levels will reveal the deficit in his later sexual performance, sexual preferences and sexual fantasies. He will be incapable of full orgastic experience in adolescent or adult life.

The care that one takes in aiding the child's potential for development in each of the psychosexual stages is inseparable from the style of child-rearing in all other aspects of living. The healthy mother is alive to her infant's oral needs and satisfies them as completely as possible. She is also in tune with the meaning of her baby's cries and responds to each appropriately, caring when care is called for, teaching the earliest lessons in democratic social structure when the cry implies imperial command. She has determined (and is at peace with the decision) that she must sacrifice some of her personal goals in the period of her child's dependency. She is prepared to be his almost constant company, playmate, instructor and satisfaction supplier. The healthy father will want to join her in this endeavor. Their interaction will be based on the premise that the more the child's needs are met, the more completely he will grow, recognizing that the need to know the limits of acceptable behavior is an important part of what he wants to know.

The contactless mother will raise her child according to a preordained plan. She will not brook interference from the child's contrary-mindedness at any point. She will find little use in referring to the child in determining her procedure. Raising her child is neither a communal adventure, a mutual learning experience nor a dialogue. It is simply a chain of command; and she is certain of who is higher on that ladder. Another variety of contactless mother is so harried and overwhelmed by life that raising a child is simply an added burden that increases her distraught lunges at solutions. There is no philosophy, no concept, only the desperate, disorganized attempt to cope.

The cultist mother pays attention to her child, but only as far as the cult doctrine reaches. Lacking balance in her own life, she is unaware that the excesses to which she carries her "belief" are creating a state of disequilibrium in her child. The extent of the damage that is inflected on the child is a function of the absurdity of the doctrine and the tenacity with which it is held. The mother who thrusts her nipple into the child's mouth every time he squeaks will raise a demanding but, to some extent, well-fed child. The mother who fails to put a gate on the stairway because she believes that, in falling repeatedly, her one-year-old will learn to avoid the danger, will raise an insecure wreck.

The abiding principle of healthy child-rearing is that the satisfaction of the dependent child's needs will lead to the most complete person and the one who most rapidly becomes independent. There are many unanswered questions relating to child development, and probably many pertinent unasked questions. We are not yet free enough of our own structural defects to observe and respond to our children with invariable objectivity. But at least we know that we must look to them and learn.

Chapter 11
Of Kreiselwelle and Cimbaloms
(A Ramble Along A Spiral Path)

After two-and-a-half years of conscientious therapy, Dennis smiled. We had gone through many hard times. I had dinned his ears with anger and frustration at his passive-aggressive maneuvers. I had jogged him unconscionably in the attempt to elicit honest responses. In his turn, he had frequently berated me for "monomaniacal" preoccupation with whatever therapeutic maneuver I was engaged in at that time, belittled the therapy when nothing happened in a session and attempted to rationalize away whatever did occur. And now, after a lifetime of pouting, he was smiling at me.

We are driving on a road in Kenya. In the distance a tall, bare acacia tree is leafed with baboons. As our car approaches, the leafy troop melts down the tree trunk and spills across the road, retreating from us.

Why had my mind recovered that scene at the moment Dennis's face opened? The association was in the movement. The face came alive and moved into the smile with the same subtle flow as the baboon troop descending from the tree. The similitude of the flow of energy in biological organisms had jogged the memory from Africa. I might also have remembered a bird spreading its wings, an insect's antennae teasing the wind for signals or the movement of my cat's ears at an unusual sound.

The free functional movement of energy through an organism is always beautiful and communicative. Artificial inhibition of that movement (which must be distinguished from natural inhibition, such as temporarily delayed action -- as in stalking animals) is always ugly. Tight lips are hideous and so is the stance of a dog disciplined to viciousness.

A person can train himself to inhibit the free flow of energy through his body. We can never train to free flow; that must be nurtured, elicited. We can learn to produce stage laughs, polite smiles and modulated voices. We can never learn spontaneous laughter, warm smiles or the thrilled voice. We can send our gawky daughters to ballet class, and by removing the inhibitions to movement, this learning can make them less awkward -- but not graceful.

Grace is a curve that moves us -- unless we block it. When we are free we can submit to it. Then the precise word occurs to us when we write, the song sings in our head when we compose, our body keeps surprising us as we dance. To be graceful is to be alive to the unknown within and without, to flow-in and flow-out as we are moved, sentient to the "different drummer" who beats a dance of spirals.

Our telescopes extend to deepest space and bring back images of spiral galaxies. Our planet circles the sun, marking a spiral path as it follows the sun, which is also moving in space. A blade of grass spirals from earth to the atmosphere to grow toward the sun. There is something special, quintessential as energy distributes mass in spiral configurations through space and time. Our ability to respond to the curl of energy within and without us is blocked by armoring, which makes us angular, stiff, straight. It keeps us from our curve, from the energetic pool of our inspiration.

To avoid misunderstanding, we must add that, though submission to the spinning wave of energy (Kreiselwelle) in oneself is the source of inspiration, it is not the stuff of great works. One does not compose by merely thrilling to the universe. The tools of the craft are indispensable; in the case of music composition, they would be the grasp of theory, harmony, counterpoint, and the gift to create song. In those blessed with inspiration, the acquisition of the tools often comes easier, as if a favorable wind pursues them. In other cases, artists become accomplished in their crafts through unusual diligence; here the following wind keeps them riveted to their course.[30]

One can best appreciate the communicative quality of an emotionally alive mind by comparing its work to a work produced by computer or by chance. We can find musical works, for example, created by successive throws of dice. Such compositions are sometimes boring, sometimes intellectually intriguing, but never moving. They

---

[30] Penfield, W., M.D., *The American Scholar,* Copyright, 1974.

[1] Discussing the qualities of the human "mind" in reference to what we have learned of the qualities of the brain through mechanistic studies, the eminent neurologist Dr. Wilder Penfield writes: "By listening to patients as they describe an experimental flashback, one can understand the complexity and efficiency of the reflex coordinating an integrative action of the brain. In it, the automatic computer and the highest brain-mechanism play interactive roles, selectively inhibitory and purposeful.

[2] Does this explain the action of the mind? Can reflex action in the end account for it? After years of studying the emerging mechanism within the brain, my own answer is 'no.' Mind comes into action and goes out of action with the highest mechanism, it is true. But the mind is peculiar. It has energy. The form of that energy is different from that of neuronal potentials that travel the axone pathways. There I must leave it."

don't breathe. No matter how one manipulates the structure by altering tempi or dynamics, one cannot make the music into an emotionally compelling experience. On the other hand, the work of an inspired composer in the hands of true artists can be varied according the breath of the performer, and each time the attentive listener will be carried by the same sweep that impels the performer. Thus, for example, Scarlatti sonatas may be performed by the late Clara Haskil[31] in an intensely concentrated performance or with a Hungarian passion by Aladar Racz[32] on the cimbelom, and each performance is valid and stirring. This intensely moving artistic experience does not occur solely in the classical art forms. One can hear the echoes of the endless spiral in the voices of Billie Holiday and Peggy Lee, for example. It is not the style that is particularly significant; it is "the awful daring of the moment's surrender." Momentary possession by the awesome wind of cosmic energy is the catalyst not only of artistic creativity but of important scientific insight.

There is a widespread popular misunderstanding that the mere application of scientific methodology and inductive reasoning to any scientific problem yields significant results. In this schema, the experiment is the source of the knowledge. This is a cozy view of science, for it implies that we already have the basic tools for all future discoveries, and that all that is lacking for the infinite increase of our knowledge is the number and ingenuity of the experimental designers.

A review of the history of scientific discovery unmasks this concept. The grand discovery is often preceded by the perception of a problem in an area where none had ever been discerned. Even in those cases in which the discovery follows a series of observations which build to a new, overpowering conclusion (a model of scientific operation), the moment of insight belongs to mind, rather than method. And against the ideal theoretical model there stand the many instances where great scientific minds refused to recognize obvious conclusions. Koestler[33] has documented this phenomenon, which he calls "snowblindedness" in fascinating detail. "Kepler...nearly threw away the elliptic (planetary) orbits; for almost three years he held the solution in his hands -- without seeing it. His conscious mind refused to accept the 'cart load of dung' which the underground had cast up."

---

[31] *The Art of Clara Haskil*, Westminster XU-R18301.
[32] *Aladar Racz at the Cimbalom*, Bartok Records No. 929.
[33] Koestler, Arthur, *The Act of Creation*, Macmillan Co., N.Y., 1964.

Galileo refused to believe in the reality of the comets which he observed, and assumed that they were optical illusions because they moved in long elliptical orbits rather than in perfect circles. Perfect circles were the only celestial movements he was prepared to acknowledge.

On the other hand, Koestler[34] reveals instances in which the correct conclusion was attained despite mathematical error or faulty logic, as if the scientist were bound to arrive at his destination despite his misdirection because he knew the answer.

The hypothesis, not the experiment, propels man's understanding. The experiment is the acid in which the validity of the hypothesis is tested. The function of the experiment is to save us from false hypotheses and theories. Moreover, contrary to casual assumption, the most valuable theory, as Popper[35] has shown, is not the one which most readily yields to easy experimental confirmation. He says, "It is easy to obtain confirmations, or verifications, for nearly every theory -- if we look for confirmations. Confirmations should count only if they are the result of risky predictions; that is to say, if unenlightened by the theory in question, we should have expected an event which was incompatible with the theory -- an event which would have refuted the theory."

Once again, as in artistic creativity, we are faced with the productive ferment of risk, curvature -- as opposed to the straight line. The creative scientist must descend into the same frightening, risky, dark night as the creative artist to seize his inspiration. Obviously, this descent is the necessary, but insufficient, fact of creativity, else we should have hordes of schizophrenic creators. To have mastered the vocabulary in which the problem is stated, to be familiar with the tools, to be occupied and preoccupied with the attempt at solution, are usually indispensable prerequisites also. Even then, we do not know why some make the connection and some do not.

To underscore the essential oneness of all creativity, whether artistic or scientific, we have the evidence of the increasing use in science of the vocabulary of aesthetics. There are "elegant" mathematical demonstrations and "beautiful" proofs (which, by the way are an index to the scientist of the probable experimental validation of

[34] Koestler, Arthur, *The Sleep Walkers.*
[35] Popper, Karl R., *Conjectures Refutations*, *The Growth of Scientific Knowledge*, Basic Books, N.Y., 1962.

his solution). There is even a class of subatomic particles that displays "a combination of properties termed charm."[36]

The consonance of creative processes in enterprises as various as the arts and sciences follows a pattern that Reich discerned in many realms of existence, particularly in those dealing with nature. Whereas from the distal (the farthest away) end, science and art appear as disparate functions, when one probes for the source of each, he discovers a single root at the proximal (the closest) end. In nature one traces a confusion of twigs to a single branch, a confusion of branches to a single trunk. Opposites (or varieties) are united at their origins into a single source and thereby share identical qualities. Through a comprehension of the process of branching, one understands the varieties of species in terms of genus, the many brooks in terms of the rivers flowing into the sea, the manifold capillaries in terms of the circulatory system of arteries and veins, the branches in terms of the trees. The coalescence of branches unites variation and makes us understand.

Heraclitus grasped this when he wrote, "Life and death, being awake and being asleep, youth and old age, all these are the same. . . for the one turned round is the first. . . The path that leads up and the path that leads down are the same path... For God all things are beautiful and good and just, but men assume some things to be unjust, and others to be just."

Commenting on this passage, Karl Popper[37] says, "Thus in truth (and for God) the opposites are identical; it is only to man that they appear as non-identical. And all things are one -- they are all part of the process of the world, the everlasting fire."

The simultaneous antithesis and functional identity of opposites was regarded as a priori knowledge by Reich.[38] He fashioned it into a radical conceptual tool for investigating living nature. By assuming that there is an identifying, common functioning principle, he leads us to a level beyond that of the phenomenon we are investigating. Reich conducts us from the capillary end -- points of natural observation -- toward the heart of nature. Reich believes it is significant that the conceptual tool with which he investigates the natural order conforms to the configuration of that order.

---

[36] *The New York Times,* November 17, 1974.
[37] Popper, Karl R., *Conjectures Refutation, The Growth of Scientific Knowledge,* Basic Books, N.Y., 1962.
[38] Reich, W., *Ether, God and Devil.*

164

He regards it not only as a useful tool, but as the only valid means of obtaining knowledge of certain living qualities (as contrasted to mechanistic qualities of natural phenomena).

The reader embarked with us on our ramble along an allegedly spiral path. He followed us around the curve of open emotion and unarmored movement, past the swirls of energy cyclones into which we dip to receive the power of creativity. But now that we are entering into a discussion of branched configurations, he may wonder about its relatedness to spirals and curves. A few linear maps should serve

If we grasp our original spiral

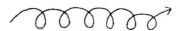

and stretch it by tugging on the ends, we arrive at the oscillating curve

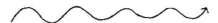

This is the curve of which Heraclitus speaks, in which, "the path that leads up and the path that leads down are the same path." What we have done in the final step is to freeze a moment conceptually on the up and down path, and instead of viewing it as

we have chosen to represent the opposing points in abstract form

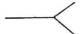

rather than in its living curve. Now, let us proceed.

The principle of cause and effect enables us to comprehend mechanistic events. But cause, effect, mathematical calculations, chemistry, physics -- though they enable us to understand particular mechanical aspects of natural functioning, such as the workings of an enzyme in the digestive process -- always fail to grasp the vital quality of an organism's path through life. An organism is obviously not merely the mechanical sum of its organs, nor are the organs simply mechanical-chemical parts sitting by waiting for messages from the brain. The organs are at once independent (which is indicated by the fact that in suitable conditions they can continue to exist outside the body), and dependent in the sense that their independent potential is subordinated to the uses of the organism-as-a-whole in natural circumstances. In orgonomic functional thinking 'cause' is replaced by common functioning principle (CFP) and 'effect' by variations.

The usefulness of the functional method will become clear if we first consider the traditional approaches to the relationship between the mind and body:

1) Whatever is psychological flows from physical underpinnings. Only the organic considerations, are significant. A recurrent theme in medicine, this view is currently ascendant in the psychiatric world. The assumption that doctors will find the proper drug or physical process with which to treat each specific psychiatric disorder is the abiding article of faith. Advocates of this view make much of the ability of the major tranquilizers to quiet the troublesome schizophrenics, of the minor tranquilizers to blanket anxiety and of lithium to decrease recurrent attacks of mania. The fact that few of the improved patients function as complete human beings is not mentioned in the excitement of apparent progress.

2). The spiritual is the source of all that is physical. Whether it is called Prana or Elan Vital, or 'divine energy,' it alone is real; the physical is hardly more than an obstacle to getting back to where essence is. This view is also increasingly popular but not in medical circles. It is the doctrine of the young evangelical religious and the characterologic mystics.

3) Body and mind are separate spheres whose only relatedness is that they occur within the same body. Some who do not wish to concern themselves with the problem entertain this position by default. But far too much evidence exists of the mutual effects of soma and psyche to entertain with much vigor a credo of parallel lines.

4) Psyche and soma are merely different aspects of the same phenomenon. This view predominates among those who work in

psychosomatics. Of the four attempts to understand the mind-body problem, the last is by far the most acceptable.

Yet Reich notes that this view fails as an explanation. It emphasizes identity to the exclusion of antithesis. It leaves no place for the purely organic consideration of, say, a liver cell qua liver cell under a microscope, or the investigation of an obsession as a purely psychological phenomenon. While it rightly makes the point of identity of psyche and soma (in reference to a common functioning principle), it ignores a fact which is apparent -- psyche is not soma. Though they are interdependent, they are not interchangeable.

The functional view is that psyche and soma are simultaneously identical and antithetical with regard to the CFP, a common bioenergetic source of energy. This perspective allows for the identity in the functions, but it also asserts that in some areas psyche and soma work autonomously. This statement is represented diagramatically.

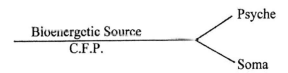

This resolution of the problem not only satisfies all contingencies of the relationship of body and mind; it is also consistent with the natural order, in which the unitary branches into variations, each of which then branches into its own variations.

The consonance of processes throughout all of nature is an abiding principle of Reich's thought. He understands the energy-discharge function of the orgasm when he recognizes that it part of the same process of biological pulsation that he observed in the ameba and the jellyfish. He regards the idea that the human animal is as a unique creation, different in any other way than as variation from the rest of the animal kingdom, as a preposterous conceit. In the same search for consistency of process throughout the universe of nature, he is led to the discovery of the function of superimposition[39] in creation. His starting point is sexual union in the biological realm. Here, two individual systems of energy flow and, because of mutual attraction, converge. The superimposition and merger results in a sharp curvature in the path of flow. This is an abstract description of sexual union, free emotion,

[39] Reich, W., *Cosmic Superimposition,* Orgone Institute Press, Maine, 1951.

psychology, culture and a host of other factors that are involved in the actual genital embrace. The virtue of such an abstraction is that it exposes the ribbing of the phenomenon, which might otherwise be concealed by flesh and clothing. Superimposition is represented diagramatically as

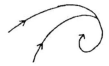

With this formulation in mind, Reich recalls his observations in the dark, metal-lined orgone-energy observation rooms where he had spent hours and days observing individual spiraling streams converges as if by attraction, and bend into a single circular path. At this point Reich makes an imaginative leap and assumes that this point of sharp curvature marks a transformation of energy into mass. The validity of this hypothesis will rest on observational and experimental confirmation or refutation in the future.

Gazing into the night skies and examining the observatory photographs of nebulae and galaxies, Reich thought that he observed the same basic process of creation in the macrocosm. The photographs of spiral nebulae suggest to him that "the creation of certain galactic systems is due to superimposition of two cosmic orgone energy streams. Most 'spiral galaxies' show two or more arms which unite toward the 'core' of the total system."

Discoveries in the future will determine whether Reich is correct in his assumption that superimposition is the common functioning principle of all creation -- from that of the transformation of primordial energy to inert mass, to the formation of galaxies in the wide heavens. Though the answer to the hypothesis is held in abeyance by our state of present ignorance, the principle of the search for consonance in biological and non-living nature is amply illustrated in the evolution of these daring conjectures.

A final word regarding orgonomic functional thought: The method does not function in the place of standard scientific procedure. It is not an armchair exercise in deciphering the world without stirring. Whether one is examining a problem from the direction of the general to the specific, or backward from the variations to the common functioning principle, the formulation can be valid only to the extent to which it is based on observation and experiment, and to which it is able to withstand future experimental refutation. Functional thought does not supplant orthodox scientific thought or procedure where orthodoxy holds valid sovereignty. But it is an invaluable aid in the investigation of that part of nature which is impermeable to conventional scientific concepts.

Our brief and very superficial investigation of orgonomic functional thought has borne us to the heavens from which we must now descend to follow the path of the infinite corkscrew of energy which moves us through life on earth.

In our discussion of the spiral path, we have failed to mention an elemental measure, the mysterious dimension -- time. When we consider that we may see tonight the light of a star emitted millions of light-years ago and long-since burnt out, the enigma of time is quite as awesome as the distance to the far quassars. When, in addition, we contemplate that time is altered by speed and "bent" by gravitational fields, our minds have entertained all the mystery they can handle.

There is a relentless quality to time that is dictated by its linear nature. Whereas events on the planet can spread to any point on the globe's surface, and emotional intensities of experience can vary from nil to overwhelming, the awareness of time can move only forward or backward.

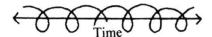

The functional experience of time is distinct from the time of the regularly ticking chronometer in the laboratory. The senile patient focuses on the time before his brain became addled; and ignoring the chronometer, he dwells in the gardens of his childhood. The malcontents conduct a large portion of their lives in the future, when revenge is theirs. Some of the oppressed bear their fate, easing their pain in the shining light of eternal time. The acutely schizophrenic lose the measure of time, or else they hew it to their particular fancy. Time rushes for the manic and drags a lead weight for the depressed.

In all lives there are accents and lacunae in time. The gravity of the time of the earliest, formative years is, in most cases, unequaled in determining the curve of one's life. In periods of high or profound emotion, when contact is keen the awareness of all the dimensions of life, including time, is more deeply impressed on our consciousness. Routine work, flattened relationships, and stereotyped patterns of living wear holes in the fabric of time. The greater the degree of armoring in an individual, the more closely the experience of time comes to resemble the flat ticking of a clock.

Time, in some cases, serves merely as the page upon which the scenario is written. In others, it is more integral to the essence of the event. It is crucial in ripening and development, in decline and death. In time profound insight becomes subverted to cliché, and the commonplace observation becomes insight. Time provides the duration for grief to spend itself and for pain to ease. The wise physician knows these uses of time, as he knows their limits.

The answers to some questions are provided only in the fullness of time. There are no instant answers to all problems, though contactless individuals sometimes function with this expectation. Some problems on the individual and societal levels are not solved. With time they become transmitted to new problems, which, in turn, are often unresolved.

Time is a significant element of the therapeutic process. Most significant changes occur in individual-evolutionary time rather than in push-button, mechanical time. The alteration of character and physical structure involve gradual reintegration of diverse systems until the new way of functioning is set. Arriving at awareness, gathering the will to risk change, accustomizing oneself to new sensations, emotions, energies -- all these require their own time.

The time of individual therapy often transcends the present and reaches into generations. One of the very satisfying aspects of the work is the knowledge that the work on the patient touches the lives of his children, an, in turn, of theirs.

In terms of our temporal existence and progress, we creep forward at a maddeningly dilatory pace. The question whether we shall succeed in freeing ourselves from our armor before the species deteriorates is unanswerable. But, given the strength of the life force, it is not unreasonable to assume that in some time, if not we, then the next more highly evolved species will live unarmored in the earth. But life will not sit, rocking in a chair, awaiting evolution. For wherever emotion (deepest self) is repressed, it will strain, no matter how distortedly, to make itself manifest. Wherever a body segment is armored, it will carry the germ of a memory of having pulsated.

Psychologie

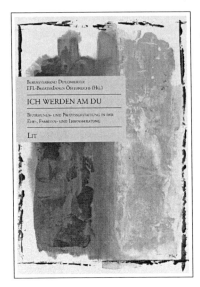

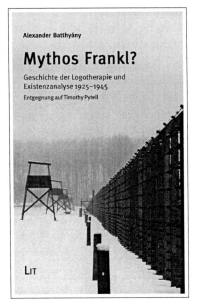

Berufsverband Diplomierter EFL-
BeraterInnen Österreichs (Hg.)
Ich werden am Du
Beziehungs- und Prozessgestaltung in der
Ehe-, Familien- und Lebensberatung
Einander zu beraten, ist eine der ältesten zwischen-
menschlichen Aktivitäten. „Der Mensch wird am
Du zum Ich", sagt Martin Buber und bietet damit
Inspiration für den Titel und den roten Faden durch
das Buch. Ehe-, Familien- und Lebensberatung ver-
steht sich als Kompetenzforum für psychosoziale
Anliegen und Krisensituationen. Sie orientiert sich
an der Problemlösung und wird auf der Basis einer
unterstützenden Beziehung durchgeführt. Die Bei-
träge bieten einen Überblick über die Entwicklung
in Österreich. Sie definieren, ohne auszugrenzen,
spüren einer beruflichen Identität nach und sind damit ein vielfältiger, aktueller, methodischer Fundus
für BeraterInnen und Interessierte.
Bd. 42, 2008, 360 S., 29,90 €, br.,
ISBN 978-3-8258-0423-7

Alexander Batthyány
Mythos Frankl?
Geschichte der Logotherapie und Existenz-
analyse 1926 – 1946. Entgegnung auf Timo-
thy Pytell
Im Frühjahr 2005 erschien das Buch „Viktor Frankl
- Ende eines Mythos?" des amerikanischen Autors
Timothy Pytell. Pytell versucht, das Leben und
Werk Viktor Frankls in einem neuen – durchwegs
negativen – Licht darzustellen. In einem Gespräch
mit dem Redakteur der Zeitschrift no:os wurde Dr.
Alexander Batthyány, Kurator des Privatarchivs von
Viktor Frankl und Herausgeber der Edition der Ge-
sammelten Werke von Vikor Frankl, um eine offene
Aussprache und detailliertere Stellungnahme zu Py-
tells Vorwürfen gebeten. Von einigen Ergänzungen
und editorischen Nachbearbeitungen abgesehen,
bringt der vorliegende Band dieses Gespräch nun in
Buchform.
Bd. 44, 2007, 112 S., 14,90 €, br.,
ISBN 978-3-8258-1032-0

LIT Verlag Berlin – Hamburg – London – Münster – Wien – Zürich
Fresnostr. 2 48159 Münster
Tel.: 0251 / 620 32 22 – Fax: 0251 / 922 60 99
e-Mail: vertrieb@lit-verlag.de – http://www.lit-verlag.de